A Case-Based Approach TO Pacemakers, ICDs, AND Cardiac Resynchronization

Volume 2

Advanced Questions for Examination Review and Clinical Practice

Edited by

Paul A. Friedman MD, FACC, FHRS | Melissa A. Rott RN

Anita Wokhlu MD | Samuel J. Asirvatham MD, FACC, FHRS

David L. Hayes MD, FACC, FHRS

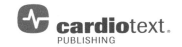

© 2011 Mayo Foundation for Medical Education and Research
First paperback edition, 2013

Cardiotext Publishing, LLC
3405 W. 44th Street
Minneapolis, Minnesota 55410 USA

www.cardiotextpublishing.com

Any updates to this book may be found at: www.cardiotextpublishing .com/titles/detail/9781935395829.

Comments, inquiries, and requests for bulk sales can be directed to the publisher at: info@cardiotextpublishing.com.

This book is intended for educational purposes and to further general scientific and medical knowledge, research, and understanding of the conditions and associated treatments discussed herein. This book is not intended to serve as and should not be relied upon as recommending or promoting any specific diagnosis or method of treatment for a particular condition or a particular patient. It is the reader's responsibility to determine the proper steps for diagnosis and the proper course of treatment for any condition or patient, including suitable and appropriate tests, medications or medical devices to be used for or in conjunction with any diagnosis or treatment.

Due to ongoing research, discoveries, modifications to medicines, equipment and devices, and changes in government regulations, the information contained in this book may not reflect the latest standards, developments, guidelines, regulations, products or devices in the field. Readers are responsible for keeping up to date with the latest developments and are urged to review the latest instructions and warnings for any medicine, equipment or medical device. Readers should consult with a specialist or contact the vendor of any medicine or medical device where appropriate.

Except for the publisher's website associated with this work, the publisher is not affiliated with and does not sponsor or endorse any websites, organizations or other sources of information referred to herein.

The publisher and the author specifically disclaim any damage, liability, or loss incurred, directly or indirectly, from the use or application of any of the contents of this book.

Unless otherwise stated, all figures and tables in this book are used courtesy of the authors.

Cover and book design: Ann Delgehausen, Trio Bookworks

Library of Congress Control Number: 2011925451
ISBN: 978-1-935395-82-9

Printed in the United States of America

7 8 9 10 11 12   24 23 22 21 20 19 18

Editors and Other Contributors

Editors

Paul A. Friedman MD, FACC, FHRS
Consultant, Division of Cardiovascular Diseases
Mayo Clinic, Rochester, Minnesota
Professor of Medicine
College of Medicine, Mayo Clinic

Melissa A. Rott RN
Heart Rhythm Services
Division of Cardiovascular Diseases
Mayo Clinic, Rochester, Minnesota

Anita Wokhlu MD
Fellow in Electrophysiology, Mayo School of Graduate
    Medical Education
College of Medicine, Mayo Clinic, Rochester, Minnesota
Assistant Professor of Medicine, College of Medicine,
    Mayo Clinic

Samuel J. Asirvatham MD, FACC, FHRS
Consultant, Divisions of Cardiovascular Diseases
    and Pediatric Cardiology
Mayo Clinic, Rochester, Minnesota
Professor of Medicine and of Pediatrics
College of Medicine, Mayo Clinic

David L. Hayes MD, FACC, FHRS
Consultant, Division of Cardiovascular Diseases
Mayo Clinic, Rochester, Minnesota
Professor of Medicine
College of Medicine, Mayo Clinic

Contributors

Craig S. Cameron MD, FACC, Oklahoma Heart Institute, Tulsa, Oklahoma (Cases 52 and 53)

Gregory A. Cogert MD, FACC, Oklahoma Heart Institute, Tulsa, Oklahoma (Cases 52 and 53)

Connie M. Dalzell RN, Mayo Clinic, Rochester, Minnesota

Joseph J. Gard MD, College of Medicine, Mayo Clinic, Rochester, Minnesota

Michael Glikson MD, FACC, FESC, Leviev Heart Center, Sheba Medical Center, Tel Hashomer, Israel (Case 54)

Michael J. Hillestad RN, Mayo Clinic, Rochester, Minnesota

Nancy Y. Lexvold RN, Mayo Clinic, Rochester, Minnesota

Madhavan Malini MBBS, College of Medicine, Mayo Clinic, Rochester, Minnesota

Marjorie L. Martin RN, Mayo Clinic, Rochester, Minnesota

David A. Sandler MD, FACC, FHRS, Oklahoma Heart Institute, Tulsa, Oklahoma (Cases 52 and 53)

Matthew J. Swale MBBS, College of Medicine, Mayo Clinic, Rochester, Minnesota

K. L. Venkatachalam MD, Mayo Clinic, Jacksonville, Florida

Tracy L. Webster RN, Mayo Clinic, Rochester, Minnesota

Preface

The book that you hold in your hands, *A Case-Based Approach to Pacemakers, ICDs, and Cardiac Resynchronization: Advanced Questions for Examination Review and Clinical Practice*, is a compilation of our favorite teaching cases that were seen at or sent to Mayo Clinic. As our device practice has grown, we have found that one of the best ways to remain current and to educate incoming physicians and nurses is the review of interesting "unknown" clinical cases. Consequently, we established a morning conference in 2008 for the purpose of presenting and discussing interesting or uniquely educational cases. Since learners ranged from cardiology fellows who were new to the device practice to experienced nurses and physicians, group discussion brought out facets of interest at all levels. Cases for this book were selected based on clinical relevance and their usefulness for illustrating general principles, practical tips, or interesting findings in device practice. Occasionally, manufacturer-specific features are discussed, but always with a goal of advancing general concepts in device management.

The cases in this book are presented as a case history, an image when pertinent, and a multiple-choice question. The answer and a detailed explanation is presented on subsequent pages. We've adopted this format to encourage the reader to think through the differential diagnosis and approach the clinical problem based on the information presented. In light of the growing use of pacemakers, defibrillators, and resynchronization devices, we are confident that readers will find this practical means of self-assessment and education useful. Although the questions are designed in a multiple-choice format that may be particularly useful for self-assessment for test-takers, they are not formally validated board questions. This book is for any individual who sees patients with implantable devices, or who will be taking an examination related to device management.

How to Use This Book

The cases generally progress from simpler to more complex, understanding that there will be individual variation in what constitutes a difficult case.

There is no table of contents because the case numbers are clearly marked at the top of each page and we specifically did not want to include in the beginning of the book a listing of the "diagnosis" for each case and therefore limit the ability for the reader to approach the cases as unknowns.

For the reader interested in reviewing a specific type of case (such as "T-wave oversensing" or "inappropriate shock"), two resources are offered. An appendix is provided that identifies the major diagnostic dilemma presented by each case, and the index will direct the reader to cases and discussions focusing on specific issues. However, we encourage readers to progress sequentially through cases as unknowns to maximize learning and interest.

This book is one of two volumes. The first volume includes introductory and intermediate cases. The second volume includes additional intermediate cases as well as advanced cases. There are more multipart cases in volume 2, to delve more deeply into important concepts.

In various electronic versions of this book, hypertext links and linked indices have been added to facilitate navigation. Also, a combined index that covers both volumes is available at www.cardiotextpublishing .com/titles/detail/9781935395447.

This text includes a collective wisdom of numerous physicians, nurses, technicians, educators, and practitioners. We are indebted to the entire Heart Rhythm services team at Mayo Clinic for identifying and discussing cases, and educating us with them. We have also benefitted greatly from friends and colleagues at other institutions who have kindly shared interesting cases with us, and permitted us to include them in this work. We are grateful for their generosity. If you come across an interesting case that you would like included in a future edition of this book, we would love to discuss it with you. E-mail addresses are listed below for that purpose. Please enjoy the cases! We look forward to your feedback and future contribution.

—Paul Friedman MD and David Hayes MD

Samuel Asirvatham: asirvatham.samuel@mayo.edu
Paul Friedman: friedman.paul@mayo.edu
David Hayes: dhayes@mayo.edu
Melissa Rott: rott.melissa@mayo.edu
Anita Wokhlu: woklhu.anita@mayo.edu

Abbreviations

A	atrial	EP	electrophysiological	PVC	premature ventricular contraction
AF	atrial fibrillation	FFRW	far-field R wave		
APC	atrial premature contraction	ICD	implantable cardioverter-defibrillator	RAO	right anterior oblique
AS	atrial sensed			RBBB	right bundle branch block
ASD	atrial septal defect	IV	intravenous	RV	right ventricle; right ventricular
AT	atrial tachycardia	J	Joules	RVOT	right ventricular outflow tract
ATP	antitachycardia pacing	LAO	left anterior oblique	SVT	supraventricular tachycardia
AV	atrioventricular	LBBB	left bundle branch block	TARP	total atrial refractory period
AVNRT	atrioventricular nodal reentrant tachycardia	LV	left ventricle; left ventricular	TENS	transcutaneous electrical nerve stimulation
		LVEF	left ventricular ejection fraction		
BBB	bundle branch block	MRI	magnetic resonance imaging	V	ventricular
CI	confidence interval	OR	odds ratio	VA	ventriculoatrial
CRT	cardiac resynchronization therapy	PA	pulmonary artery	VF	ventricular fibrillation
		PAC	premature atrial contraction	VRR	ventricular rate regulation
CT	computed tomographic	PMT	pacemaker-mediated tachycardia	VS	ventricular sensed
ECG	electrocardiogram	PVARB	postventricular atrial blanking period	VSD	ventricular septal defect
EGM	electrogram			VT	ventricular tachycardia
EMI	electromagnetic interference	PVARP	postventricular atrial refractory period		

A Case-Based Approach
to Pacemakers, ICDs, and
Cardiac Resynchronization Volume 2

Advanced Questions for Examination Review and Clinical Practice

Case 46

A 74-year-old female with a history of long QT syndrome and cardiac arrest underwent implantation of a dual-chamber defibrillator, the St. Jude Atlas +DR. The RV defibrillator lead is a Riata, which has an integrated bipolar lead. Two years later, the patient is seen in the device clinic and complains of receiving her first and only shock from the device 1 month prior. Portions of the episode are shown in Figure 46.1.

During interrogation, RV sensing and shock coil impedances are normal. The RV lead threshold is normal. The R wave today measures 8.2 mV compared to 9.0 mV at implant. Provocative maneuvers do not impact these values. The ventricular sensitivity setting was set as 0.3 mV. RV sensing parameters are as follows:

	Postsensed	Postpaced
Decay Delay	60 ms	Auto
Threshold Start	62.5%	Auto
Refractory Period	125 ms	250 ms

The patient's chest x-ray is normal. Her QT interval is 320 ms. Her potassium is 4.2 mmol/L.

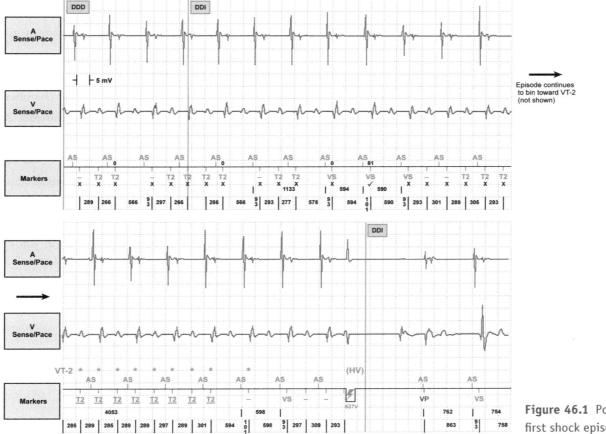

Figure 46.1 Portions of patient's first shock episode.

Q: *What would be the next most reasonable management step(s)?*

1. Correct electrolytes and initiate the patient on an antiarrhythmic agent
2. Repeat defibrillation threshold testing and consider lead revision
3. Reduce the sensitivity setting to 0.1 mV
4. Program more aggressive antitachycardic pacing therapies

46

2. Repeat defibrillation threshold testing and consider lead revision

This question requires you to recognize T-wave oversensing. Of the choices provided, the most reasonable management option is to repeat defibrillation threshold testing and consider possible lead revision for this patient with T-wave oversensing. In this case, the patient has a history of cardiac arrest. Furthermore, the R-wave amplitude measurement has diminished without a clear etiology. Her QT measures normally at follow-up and is not markedly prolonged in Figure 46.1. Repeat defibrillation threshold testing with possible lead revision represents the most appropriate management step. The ventricular lead should be revised if the safety margin for sensing ventricular fibrillation is insufficient. If the defibrillation lead is replaced, a true bipolar lead may be preferred because T-wave oversensing may be more frequent with integrated-bipolar leads (Weretka S, Michaelsen J, Becker R, et al. Ventricular oversensing: a study of 101 patients implanted with dual chamber defibrillators and two different lead systems. *Pacing Clin Electrophysiol.* 2003;26:65-70).

An annotated version of the episode is shown in Figure 46.2. On the top panel, we see multiple events labeled T2 on the ventricular marker channel, signifying that the device is binning ventricular events that count toward the VT2, or the fast VT, zone. Referring to the ventricular sensing EGM, we see that the T2 labeled events align with both the native R wave and the T wave, resulting in short R-R cycles in the 280 to

300 ms range. Hand calculation of the R-R cycle length (25 mm/s paper speed) demonstrates that the cycle length is actually 590 ms, which is more consistent with sinus tachycardia. The small gray "X's" that align with the V or T2 markers are morphology template match attempts suggesting failure to match T waves *and* intrinsic ventricular EGM to the ventricular morphology template. The checks correspond to a template match. The dashes (-) reflect a cycle length that does not count toward binning. Ventricular sense events are seen for a brief period as well. The device continues to bin events towards the VT2 zone (not shown). In the lower panel, the marker channel shows VT2, meaning that the device has binned enough events toward the VT2 zone to confirm arrhythmia. The asterisks indicate charging. During that charging, the device recon-

firms VT2 as denoted by the underlined T2 markers, and ultimately a 15-J shock is delivered.

T-wave oversensing has resulted in the inappropriate detection of VT. The amplitude of the R waves is 3.0 to 3.5 mV during this episode (from baseline to peak), which is markedly reduced from implant. This is probably the reason for the failed morphology match even for the intrinsic QRS complexes (Weretka et al. 2003). The T-wave amplitude measures 1.0 mV, 33% of the R-wave amplitude. Possible reasons for a diminution in the R-wave amplitude include electrolyte changes, tip fibrosis, infarction, infiltration, or progressive cardiomyopathy in the ventricle, a loosened set screw, or microdislodgment and macrodislodgment of the lead.

46

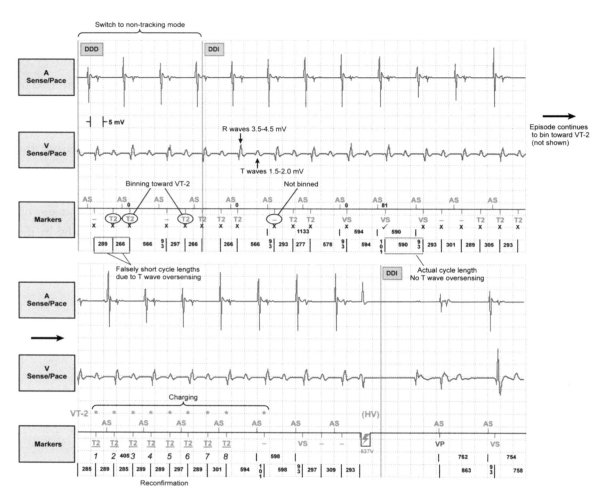

Figure 46.2 Annotated version of patient's first shock episode.

46

The patient wants to defer invasive evaluation or lead revision at this time. In general which is a reasonable set of reprogramming options in patients with this type of oversensing?

1. Lengthen the postsensing Decay Delay and increase the percentage threshold start

2. Increase the postpacing ventricular blanking period

3. Turn off SVT-VT morphology discrimination

4. All of the above

46

1. Lengthen the postsensing Decay Delay and increase the percentage threshold start

This case tests your ability to identify reprogramming options in this patient with an inappropriate shock due to T-wave oversensing.

It is helpful to think about the management of T-wave oversensing in three broad categories: postpacing, large R wave (>3 mV) in spontaneous rhythm, and small R wave (<3 mV) in spontaneous rhythm (Swerdlow CD, Friedman PA. Advanced ICD troubleshooting: part I. *Pacing clin Electrophysiol.* 2005;28(12):1322-46). Typically, the first scenario—oversensing of postpacing T waves—causes inappropriate inhibition of bradycardic pacing or delivery of antitachycardia pacing. It may be corrected by increasing the postpacing ventricular blanking period. In the second scenario in which R waves are greater than 3 mV with a large R/T ratio, reprogramming may be feasible. Some devices allow for adjusting the sensitivity threshold to a higher value. The third scenario of T-wave oversensing in the setting of low-amplitude R waves presents a more challenging situation. Options include:

- St. Jude ICDs provide a programmable Threshold Start, Decay Delay, and the postventricular refractory period designed to reduce oversensing of spontaneous T waves.

- Turning on SVT-VT morphology discrimination to "on," which may classify alternative EGMs associated with intrinsic QRS as sinus and potentially result in withholding therapy.
- If the RT and TR intervals differ sufficiently in the VT zone, the stability algorithm may be used to reject T-wave oversensing.
- Rarely, force ventricular pacing to alter the sequence of depolarization and reduce T-wave amplitude.
- Lead revision of the addition of a second pace/sense RV lead.

Management in this case was particularly difficult because the R-wave dimunition was transient. In general, R-wave amplitudes lower than 5 to 7 mV carry the risk of underdetection of VF and inappropriate shocks due to T-wave oversensing. The T-wave oversensing can often manifest when the ventricular sensitivity or gain is automatically adjusted in relation to the low-amplitude preceding R wave. Responding to this scenario by raising the minimum sensing thresholds carries the risk of undersensing native R waves, as well as underdetection of ventricular fibrillation. In this case the Decay Delay was extended from 60 to 160 ms and the threshold start was increased from 62.5% to 75.0% (Figure 46.3, adapted from Swerdlow et al. 2005). It is important to recognize that although these changes did not alter the sensitivity threshold, the window to detect VF was made effectively shorter. In some but not all reprogramming situations, repeat ventricular fibrillation induction with defibrillation threshold testing may be warranted to confirm that ventricular fibrillation is reliably detected.

Answer 2, increasing the postpacing ventricular blanking period, is incorrect because over sensing of post pacing T waves is not present. Answer 3, turning off morphology discrimination, likely would have no effect in this case but can be beneficial in patients when the intrinsic QRS matches the morphology template. Answer 4, all of the above, is incorrect.

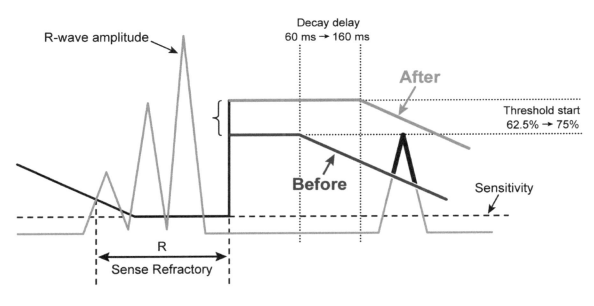

Figure 46.3 Demonstration of adjusted parameters in this patient.

Case 47

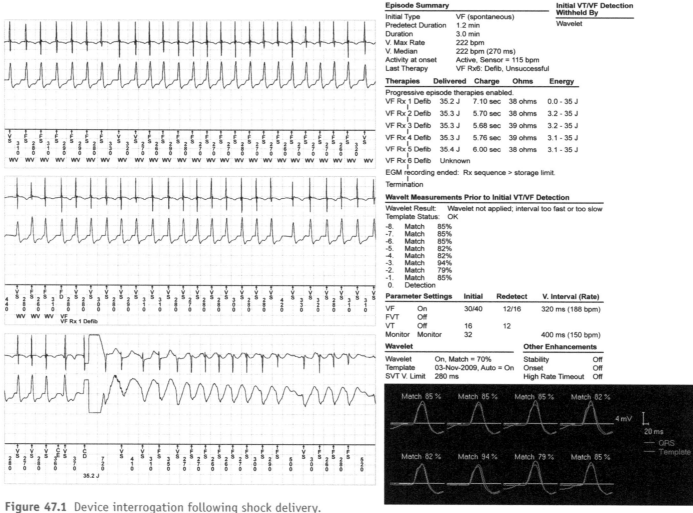

Episode Summary

Initial Type	VF (spontaneous)
Predetect Duration	1.2 min
Duration	3.0 min
V. Max Rate	222 bpm
V. Median	222 bpm (270 ms)
Activity at onset	Active, Sensor = 115 bpm
Last Therapy	VF Rx6: Defib, Unsuccessful

Initial VT/VF Detection Withheld By

Wavelet

Therapies	Delivered	Charge	Ohms	Energy
Progressive episode therapies enabled.				
VF Rx 1 Defib	35.2 J	7.10 sec	38 ohms	0.0 - 35 J
VF Rx 2 Defib	35.3 J	5.70 sec	38 ohms	3.2 - 35 J
VF Rx 3 Defib	35.3 J	5.68 sec	39 ohms	3.2 - 35 J
VF Rx 4 Defib	35.3 J	5.76 sec	39 ohms	3.1 - 35 J
VF Rx 5 Defib	35.4 J	6.00 sec	38 ohms	3.1 - 35 J
VF Rx 6 Defib	Unknown			

EGM recording ended: Rx sequence > storage limit.

Termination

Wavelt Measurements Prior to Initial VT/VF Detection

Wavelet Result:	Wavelet not applied; interval too fast or too slow
Template Status:	OK

-8.	Match	85%
-7.	Match	85%
-6.	Match	85%
-5.	Match	82%
-4.	Match	82%
-3.	Match	94%
-2.	Match	79%
-1.	Match	85%
0.	Detection	

Parameter Settings	Initial	Redetect	V. Interval (Rate)
VF	On	30/40	12/16	320 ms (188 bpm)
FVT	Off			
VT	Off	16	12	
Monitor	Monitor	32		400 ms (150 bpm)

Wavelet		Other Enhancements	
Wavelet	On, Match = 70%	Stability	Off
Template	03-Nov-2009, Auto = On	Onset	Off
SVT V. Limit	280 ms	High Rate Timeout	Off

Match 85 %   Match 85 %   Match 85 %   Match 82 %

Match 82 %   Match 94 %   Match 79 %   Match 85 %

4 mV
20 ms
— QRS
— Template

Figure 47.1 Device interrogation following shock delivery.
Episode report is shown top right. Left from top to bottom are shown near-field ventricular EGMs, far-field
ventricular EGMs, and marker channels. Bottom right is an arrhythmia episode screen shot showing morphology scores.

A 69-year-old woman received a Medtronic Secura VR ICD to prevent sudden cardiac death. Her ICD was programmed with a single zone set to detect VF if 30/40 beats were shorter than 320 ms. Wavelet was turned on with match = 70%, and AutoTemplate was on. The SVT limit was 280 ms, and stability, onset, and high-rate timeout were all off. The patient received shocks, and device interrogation is shown in Figure 47.1.

Q: *Based on this information, what is the best description of this episode?*

1. Shock due to VT
2. Shock due to morphology algorithm error
3. Shock due to tachycardia rate greater than SVT limit
4. Appropriate rejection of SVT

47

3. Shock due to tachycardia rate greater than the SVT limit

The tracing demonstrates a supraventricular tachycardia. The episode screen shot (Figure 47.2, bottom right) shows that each of the last 8 complexes prior to VF detection was listed as a morphology match, with match scores in excess of 70% (the programmed cutoff for distinguishing SVT from VT). The morphology algorithm compares a tachycardia complex to a stored template, to determine whether the complex is ventricular or supraventricular. If 6 of the last 8 complexes have a match score < 70%, the rhythm is classified as ventricular. The "WV" beneath on the marker channel in the top tracing indicates correct classification and withholding of therapy. However, the tachycardia then increases to a rate above the SVT detection limit (ie, the cycle length was shorter than the programmed SVT limit of 280 ms—see circle complex in Figure 47.2). At that point SVT-VT discrimination is withheld, rate only detection is applied, and therapy delivered. In this case, since the rhythm was supraventicular, an inappropriate shock is delivered. Note that the in-

47

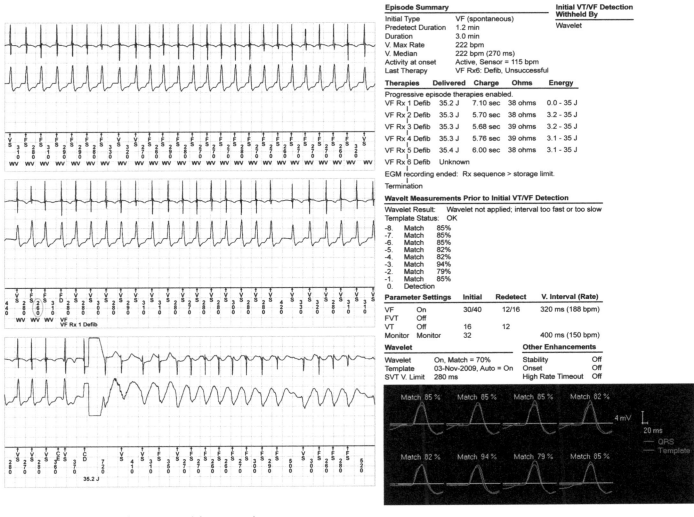

Episode Summary

Initial Type	VF (spontaneous)
Predetect Duration	1.2 min
Duration	3.0 min
V. Max Rate	222 bpm
V. Median	222 bpm (270 ms)
Activity at onset	Active, Sensor = 115 bpm
Last Therapy	VF Rx6: Defib, Unsuccessful

Initial VT/VF Detection Withheld By

Wavelet

Therapies	Delivered	Charge	Ohms	Energy
Progressive episode therapies enabled.				
VF Rx 1 Defib	35.2 J	7.10 sec	38 ohms	0.0 - 35 J
VF Rx 2 Defib	35.3 J	5.70 sec	38 ohms	3.2 - 35 J
VF Rx 3 Defib	35.3 J	5.68 sec	39 ohms	3.2 - 35 J
VF Rx 4 Defib	35.3 J	5.76 sec	39 ohms	3.1 - 35 J
VF Rx 5 Defib	35.4 J	6.00 sec	38 ohms	3.1 - 35 J
VF Rx 6 Defib	Unknown			

EGM recording ended: Rx sequence > storage limit.

Termination

Wavelt Measurements Prior to Initial VT/VF Detection

Wavelet Result: Wavelet not applied; interval too fast or too slow
Template Status: OK

-8.	Match	85%
-7.	Match	85%
-6.	Match	85%
-5.	Match	82%
-4.	Match	82%
-3.	Match	94%
-2.	Match	79%
-1.	Match	85%
0.	Detection	

Parameter Settings	Initial	Redetect	V. Interval (Rate)
VF	On	30/40	12/16	320 ms (188 bpm)
FVT	Off			
VT	Off	16	12	
Monitor	Monitor	32		400 ms (150 bpm)

Wavelet		Other Enhancements	
Wavelet	On, Match = 70%	Stability	Off
Template	03-Nov-2009, Auto = On	Onset	Off
SVT V. Limit	280 ms	High Rate Timeout	Off

Match 85 %   Match 85 %   Match 85 %   Match 82 %

4 mV
20 ms
— QRS
— Template

Match 82 %   Match 94 %   Match 79 %   Match 85 %

Figure 47.2 Same as Figure 47.1 with annotations.

47

terval histogram in Figure 47.3 shows marked variation, consistent with atrial fibrillation. In Medtronic devices the SVT limit is independently programmable, so that SVT-VT detection enhancements like morphology can be applied independent of VT/VF boundaries. However, some detection enhancements (notably stability) are not applied in the VF zone since both AF and VF may be irregular. In Boston Scientific and St. Jude Medical ICDs, detection enhancements are applied in VT but not VF zones.

Answer 1 is incorrect since VT is not present. Answer 2 is incorrect since the morphology algorithm correctly classified the rhythm, but was then no longer applied when the tachycardia intervals shortened beyond the SVT limit. Answer 4 is incorrect, since ultimately the SVT was not rejected, and a shock was delivered. Reprogramming to a faster SVT limit, or treating the patient with a rate-slowing agent (or both) may prevent future shocks. Note that multiple shocks were delivered (episode report, top right).

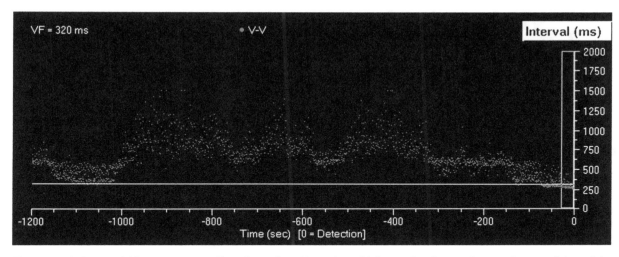

Figure 47.3 Interval histogram preceding detection. Note the widely varying intervals, consistent with atrial fibrillation. The increasing heart rate (shorter intervals) led to detection in the VF zone at a rate above the SVT limit.

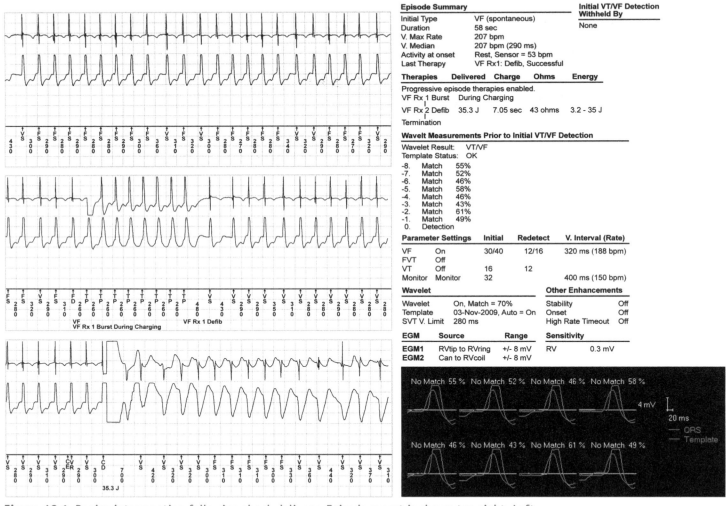

Figure 48.1 Device interrogation following shock delivery. Episode report is shown top right. Left from top to bottom are shown near-field ventricular EGMs, far-field ventricular EGMs, and marker channels. Bottom right is an arrhythmia episode screen shot showing morphology scores.

48

You look at additional tracings from the same 69-year-old woman from case 47 with a Medtronic Secura VR ICD implanted to prevent sudden cardiac death. Her ICD was programmed with a single zone set to detect VF if 30/40 beats were shorter than 320 ms. Wavelet was turned on with match = 70%, and AutoTemplate was on. The SVT limit was 280 ms, and stability, onset, and high-rate timeout were all off. The additional tracings of interest are shown in Figure 48.1.

Q: *Based on this information, what is the best description of this episode?*

1. Shock due to VT
2. Shock due to morphology algorithm error
3. Shock due to rate greater than SVT limit
4. Appropriate rejection of SVT

48

2. Shock due to morphology algorithm error

The arrhythmia in this tracing looks very similar to the one seen in case 47, with the far-field EGMs that look very similar to the case 47 EGMs, suggesting SVT. In this case, however, the morphology algorithm scores each of the last 8 complexes as "No Match" (shaded section of Episode report in Figure 48.2, and arrhythmia episode screen shot, bottom right). Note that one of the complexes has been magnified showing that the top of the EGM is trucated. This is also seen in the tracings (bottom right). Clipping of the signal by the amplifier results in EGM distortion leading morphology to misclassify SVT as VT. A side-by-side comparison of the nonclipped EGM from case 47 and the clipped EGM in this case from the same patient is shown in Figure 48.3, highlighting the EGM distortion caused by clipping. In Medtronic and St. Jude ICDs, dynamic range is programmable and should be checked at implant and at follow-ups so that the EGM fills 25% to 75% of the window. In Medtronic devices up to Protecta, the window is nominally set at +/- 8 mV. From Protecta forward, it is set at 16 mV to minimize clipping risk.

Morphology algorithms play an increasingly important role in ICD discrimination.

The general steps within a morphology discrimination algorithm are:

1. Obtain a representative ventricular EGM template during baseline rhythm.
2. Generate a quantitative representation of this template that is stored for future comparison.
3. Obtain a ventricular EGM during an unknown tachycardia and translate it into a quantitative representation.
4. Time align the ventricular EGMs for comparison.
5. Compare the degree of similarity between the quantitative representation of the unknown tachycardia to that of the reference template during baseline rhythm.
6. Classify the unknown tachycardia either as VT if the morphology is significantly different from the baseline or as SVT if the morphologies are similar.

Since the morphology of an EGM may change during lead maturation after being newly implanted, algorithms automatically acquire and update the templates periodically. Defibrillation alters the surface ECG and EGM morphology for minutes following shock delivery, so morphology algorithms are not used during redetection. There are differences in how the device manufacturers implement each of the steps of morphology detection enhancements, but all have common failure modes (Swerdlow CD, Friedman PA. Advanced ICD troubleshooting: part 1. *PACE*. 2005;28:1322-1346).

An EGM is *truncated* when its amplitude exceeds the sensing amplifier's dynamic range, as in this case. *Alignment* errors lead to misclassification of similar EGMs as different due to improper alignment. St Jude ICDs use the onset of the EGM as the point of reference for alignment. Since ICD sensing is dynamic and affected by heart rate, the point of EGM onset may vary based on the rate at the time of acquisition, leading

48

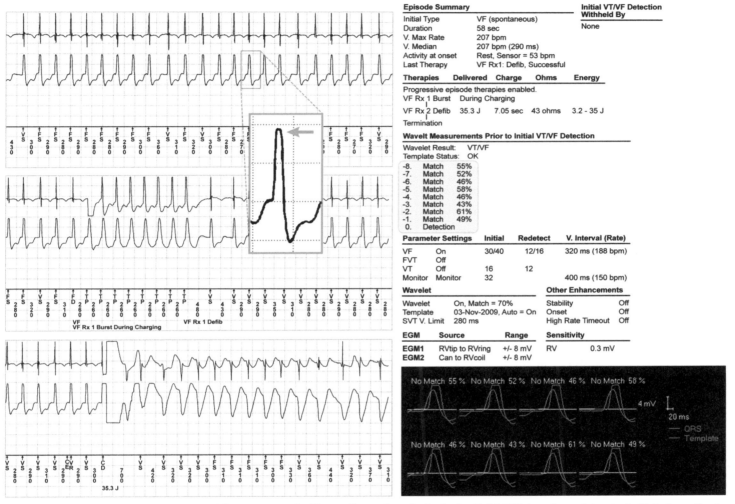

Episode Summary

Initial Type	VF (spontaneous)
Duration	58 sec
V. Max Rate	207 bpm
V. Median	207 bpm (290 ms)
Activity at onset	Rest, Sensor = 53 bpm
Last Therapy	VF Rx1: Defib, Successful

Initial VT/VF Detection Withheld By

None

Therapies   Delivered   Charge   Ohms   Energy

Progressive episode therapies enabled.
VF Rx 1 Burst   During Charging

VF Rx 2 Defib   35.3 J   7.05 sec   43 ohms   3.2 - 35 J

Termination

Wavelet Measurements Prior to Initial VT/VF Detection

Wavelet Result: VT/VF
Template Status: OK

-8.	Match	55%
-7.	Match	52%
-6.	Match	46%
-5.	Match	58%
-4.	Match	46%
-3.	Match	43%
-2.	Match	61%
-1.	Match	49%
0.	Detection	

Parameter Settings   Initial   Redetect   V. Interval (Rate)

VF	On	30/40	12/16	320 ms (188 bpm)
FVT	Off			
VT	Off	16	12	
Monitor	Monitor	32		400 ms (150 bpm)

Wavelet

Wavelet	On, Match = 70%
Template	03-Nov-2009, Auto = On
SVT V. Limit	280 ms

Other Enhancements

Stability	Off
Onset	Off
High Rate Timeout	Off

EGM   Source   Range   Sensitivity

EGM1	RVtip to RVring	+/- 8 mV	RV	0.3 mV
EGM2	Can to RVcoil	+/- 8 mV		

No Match 55 %   No Match 52 %   No Match 46 %   No Match 58 %

4 mV

20 ms

QRS
Template

No Match 46 %   No Match 43 %   No Match 61 %   No Match 49 %

Figure 48.2 Same as Figure 48.1 but with accents to facilitate discussion. A single far-field EGM is enlarged (center). Note how the top of the EGM is clipped (arrow). Clipping caused misclassification as VT. It can be corrected by adjusting the EGM's dynamic range.

48

to misalignment. In Medtronic ICDs, the tallest peak of the EGM is for alignment; peak distortion due to truncation or rate-related changes may lead to misalignment. Boston Scientific ICDs assess morphology by a vector timing and correlation algorithm that utilizes the near-field EGM, which is generally sharper (greater slew) for alignment, and then following alignment compares features of the far-field EGM. (Swerdlow 2005) Alignment errors can occur if there are changes in the near-field EGM.

An *inaccurate template* will lead to inappropriate classification of SVT as VT. Ectopy and intermittent bundle branch block that occur during template acquisition can lead to its inaccuracy. Since the morphology of the ventricular EGM can also change as the lead matures following implant, the inability to acquire updated templates due to frequent ectopy or absence of an intrinsic rhythm may lead to inaccuracies. If periodic templates cannot be acquired, morphology should not be used until lead maturation is complete, typically around 3 months postimplant.

Rate-related *aberrancy* may result in misclassification of SVT as VT. If it occurs reproducibly, automatic template updating should be turned off and a template acquired while pacing in the AAI mode at a rate sufficient to acquire the aberrancy. Since the degree of aberrancy may be variable during irregular SVTs such as atrial fibrillation, reducing the fraction of EGM required to exceed the match threshold (from 5 of 8 to 4 of 8 in St. Jude ICDs) may ameliorate the problem without impairment of VT detection.

SVT *soon after shocks* may lead to misclassification due to postshock EGM distortion. While morphology is not used during redetection, if an episode during which a shock is delivered is terminated and a new episode develops within several minutes, residual EGM distortion may be present during detection.

Pectoral myopotentials do not result in shocks in the absence of tachycardia, since the pulse generator is not used as a sensing electrode in the rate-detecting channel. However, pectoral myopotentials can lead to inappropriate detection of SVT as VT by distorting the far-field EGM during SVT, leading to mismatch. This may be seen during sinus tachycardia caused by exercise. Medtronic (nominally) and Boston Scientific ICDs use the far-field EGM during morphology discrimination, whereas St. Jude ICDs use the near-field EGM, and thus are not susceptible to pectoral myopotential oversensing.

Answer 1 is incorrect since there is no evidence that VT is present, and there is clear evidence of EGM clipping, suggesting morphology algorithm error. Answer 3 (shock due to rate greater than SVT limit) is incorrect because the rate of the VT was 290 ms, and the SVT limit is set for 280 ms. The SVT limit withholds application of SVT-VT discriminators when the programmed SVT limit rate is exceeded (ie, cycle length is shorter than the programmed limit). Since the VT cycle length (290 ms) was *longer* than the SVT limit, the morphology algorithm was applied. Answer 4 is incorrect since SVT was not rejected, but was in fact treated.

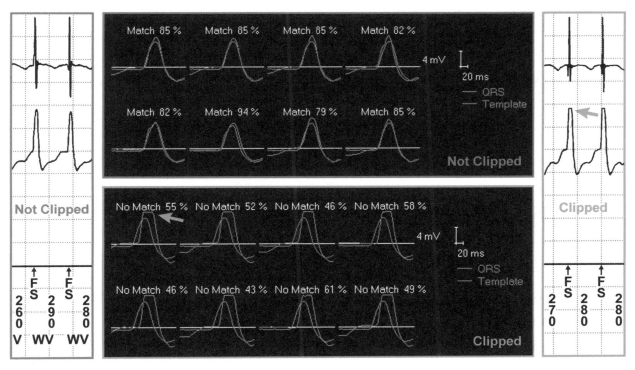

Figure 48.3 A side-by-side comparison of nonclipped (left and top center) and clipped (bottom center and right) EGMs from the same patient. Since the Medtronic ICD uses the EGM peak for alignment, clipping of the signal ("truncation") can lead to misclassification by 2 mechanisms: EGM distortion or misalignment of tachycardia with template.

Case 49

A 76-year-old woman calls the device clinic for a routine transtelephonic transmission. She had a DDDR pacemaker implanted 3 years earlier. Pacemaker function has been normal to date.

Device settings:
- Mode: DDDR
- Pacing rate: 60 to 120 bpm
- PVARP: 310 ms
- AVI: dynamic AV delay on with maximum 250 ms, minimum 180 ms
- Atrial output: 5 V at 0.4 ms
- Ventricular output: 5 V at 0.3 ms

A nonmagnet transmission was obtained (Figure 49.1).

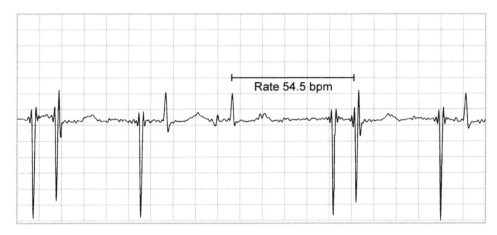

Figure 49.1 Patient's nonmagnet transmission.

Q: *The ventricular rate of 54.5 bpm is a result of which of these?*

1. Ventricular oversensing
2. Fallback response
3. Modified atrial-based timing
4. Rate smoothing

49

3. Modified atrial-based timing

All pacemakers have a defined "timing" system. The timing system may be ventricular-based or atrial-based, and modifications of both timing systems are common.

A ventricular-based timing system is one in which the VA interval is fixed (Figure 49.2). A ventricular sensed event occurring during the VA interval resets the timer, causing it to begin again. A ventricular sensed event occurring during the AV interval terminates the AV interval and initiates the VA interval. If there is intact conduction through the AV node following an atrial pacing stimulus such that the AR interval (atrial stimulus to sensed R wave) is shorter than the programmed AV interval, the resulting paced rate will accelerate by a small amount.

In contrast to a ventricular-based system, in an atrial-based pacemaker timing system, the AA interval is fixed. As long as lower-rate-limit pacing is stable, there is no discernible difference between the two timing systems. In a system with atrial-based timing, a sensed R wave that occurs during the AV interval inhibits the ventricular output but does not alter the basic AA timing (Figure 49.3). Hence, the rate stays at the programmed lower rate limit during effective single-chamber atrial pacing. When a ventricular premature beat is sensed during the atrial escape interval, the timers also are reset, but it is the AA interval rather than the atrial escape interval that is reset.

In this patient the observed VV interval is longer than the programmed lower rate limit. As long as the ventricle is being paced, the escape interval is timed from one V event to the next. Whenever a sensed V event occurs, ie, intrinsic AV conduction before the AV delay elapses, the timing base switches from ventricular-based timing to atrial-based

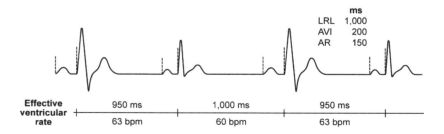

Figure 49.2 Ventricular-based timing.

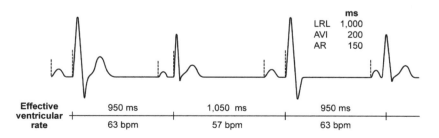

Figure 49.3 Atrial-based timing.

timing. This ensures accurate (atrial) pacing rates even during intrinsic AV conduction.

The difference that explains the rate changes is the interval between the programmed AVI and the AR interval.

Extension = AVI – AR

In this specific pacemaker, the timing system in effect when the device is in the DDDR or DDIR mode is a modified atrial-based timing system (Figure 49.4).

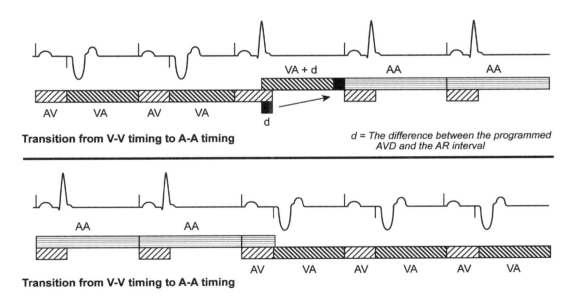

Figure 49.4 Modified atrial-based timing system. As long as the ventricle is being paced, the escape interval is timed from one V event to the next. Whenever a sensed V event occurs, ie, intrinsic AV conduction before the AV delay elapses, the timing base switches from ventricular-based timing to atrial-based timing. This ensures accurate pacing rates even during intrinsic AV conduction. From Insignia I Ultra Technical Manual; Figure 6-2; Boston Scientific, with permission.

49

More specifically, in Figure 49.5:

- LRL: 60 bpm = 1000 ms
- Interval noted on TTM = 54.5 bpm = 1100 ms, ie, 100 ms longer than programmed lower rate limit (LRL)
- Programmed AVI: 250 ms

The longest potential difference would be if the V sensed event occurred simultaneously with AS or AP (ie, AR = 0); extension = AVI – AR

For purposes of calculation, longest AVI = 250 ms and the effective VV interval is 100 ms longer than the programmed LRL; therefore AR was 150 ms

Extension (100) = AVI (250) – AR (150)

This would not represent "fallback response," (answer 2) which is defined as a programmable upper rate response of some dual-chamber pacemakers. Fallback occurs when an atrial tachyarrhythmia results in a mode switch to a nontracking mode. Rather than the ventricular rate abruptly falling to the lower rate limit (or sensor-driven rate) from the high rate at the time of mode switch, it gradually falls back to the lower rate to minimize symptoms. In this tracing there is no atrial tachyarrhythmia and no gradually prolonging intervals ("falling back") to suggest this diagnosis.

Rate smoothing is an algorithm that introduces a pacing impulse earlier than expected to minimize cycle length variation that may occur with any premature complex. In this tracing, the finding is that the ventricular paced complex appears *delayed, not early.* This excludes rate smoothing, answer 4, as a possibility. The most aggressive rate smoothing programmable option is usually 12%, ie, if decremental rate smoothing was programmed on the most, the cycle length decrement would be 12% of the preceding interval.

Oversensing (answer 1) should always be considered when the lower rate limit is violated with a longer interval, but intervals would usually be highly variable and extremely unlikely to fit the expected modified atrial timing exactly. Additionally, oversensing is often seen in the setting of baseline noise or artifact to suggest the presence of noise, although this finding may be absent via transtelephonic recordings.

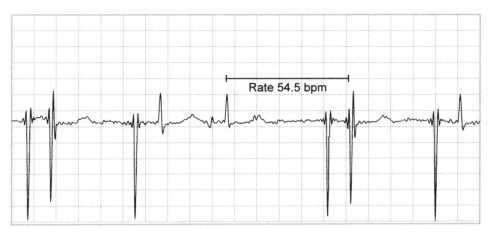

Figure 49.5 Patient's tracing. (Same as Figure 49.1.)

Case 50

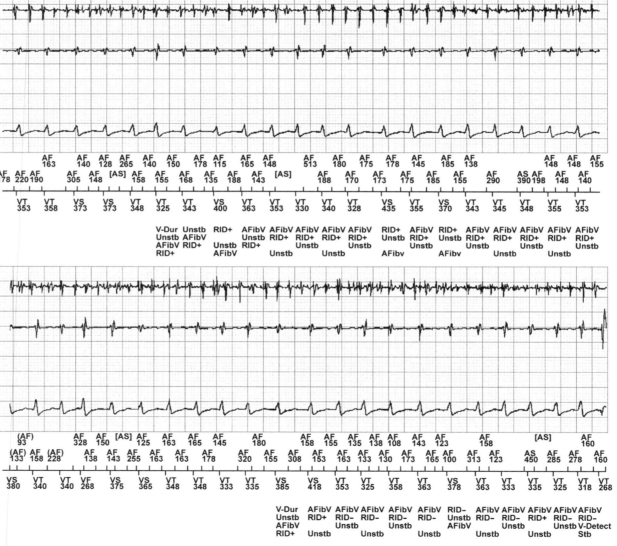

Figure 50.1 Detection preceding shock delivery. From top to bottom are shown the atrial, rate sensing (near-field ventricular), and shock (far-field ventricular) EGMs. Below those are the markers. Top panel: untreated episode. Bottom panel: treated episode.

A 73-year-old woman with an ischemic cardiomyopathy received a Teligen 100 implantable defibrillator. She presents with a shock and her device is interrogated. The shock charge time was 5.7 seconds, the lead impedance 35 ohms, and the polarity initial.

Figure 50.1 shows the tracing from the device interrogation demonstrating the detection that immediately preceded shock delivery (bottom panel). Multiple similar episodes without shock had also been seen (top panel).

Q: *Based on this interrogation, what is the most likely cause of the shock?*

1. Ventricular tachycardia that occurred during atrial fibrillation
2. AF inappropriately detected as ventricular tachycardia
3. AF that accelerates into the VF zone
4. Lead fracture

50

2. AF inappropriately detected as ventricular tachycardia

The actual rhythm is AF. The ventricular rate is rapid, in the VT zone, resulting in "VT" markers. Once 8 out of 10 ventricular events exceed the VT detection rate, a duration timer is started. Once the duration timer is met (nominally 2.5 sec in the VT zone), the device proceeds to therapy delivery. Note that duration is met with the occurrence of the complex in the red box shown in Figure 50.2, with the marker "V-Dur" underneath. Despite completion of the duration interval, therapy is initially withheld due to the detection enhancement (Rhythm ID), which initially correctly classifies the rhythm as supraventricular. Rhythm ID initially compares the atrial and ventricular rates, the EGM morphology, and the interval stability to classify an arrhythmia (Figure 50.3). The "Unstb" marker indicates QRS interval variability consistent with AF. The "RID+" marker indicates that the morphology analysis indicates supraventricular tachycardia as well.

With the blue-circled complex the marker changes to "RID–." This indicates that the morphology is now considered different from the baseline template, and the device would diagnose VT base on morphology.

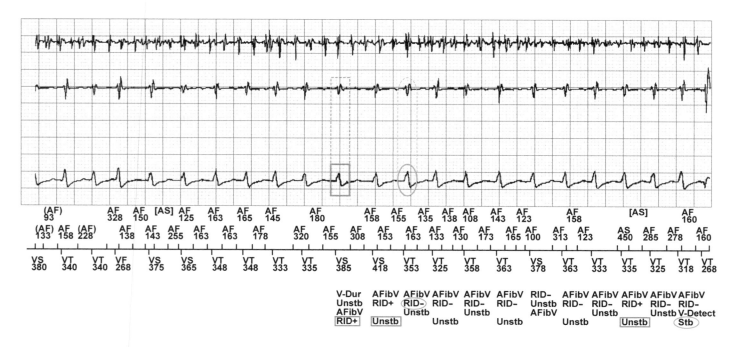

Figure 50.2 Same as bottom panel in Figure 50.1 but with annotations added.

50

However, since Rhythm ID also assesses interval stability, and the overall rhythm remains unstable ("Unstb"), therapy is withheld at this point (Figure 50.3).

Note that the actual change in the morphology of the complexes in the rectangle and circle is minimal. During AF slight changes in morphology can often occur due to longitudinal dissociation (activation of different fibers in the His-Purkinje system). These morphological changes are usually much smaller than the gross distortions seen with rate-related bundle branch block (aberrancy). The algorithm in this device

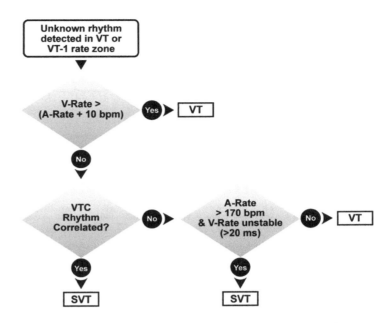

Figure 50.3 Rhythm ID algorithm. Initially, a comparison between atrial and ventricular rate is used to classify the rhythm. If SVT is declared in the first step, then the morphology (VTC = vector timing correlation, a morphology analysis) is assessed. If the rhythm's morphology does not match the baseline template, possibilities include aberrant SVT or VT. In the last step, assessment of the atrial rate (to confirm ongoing AF) and interval stability is used to differentiate VT (stable intervals) from SVT (unstable, or variable intervals).

50

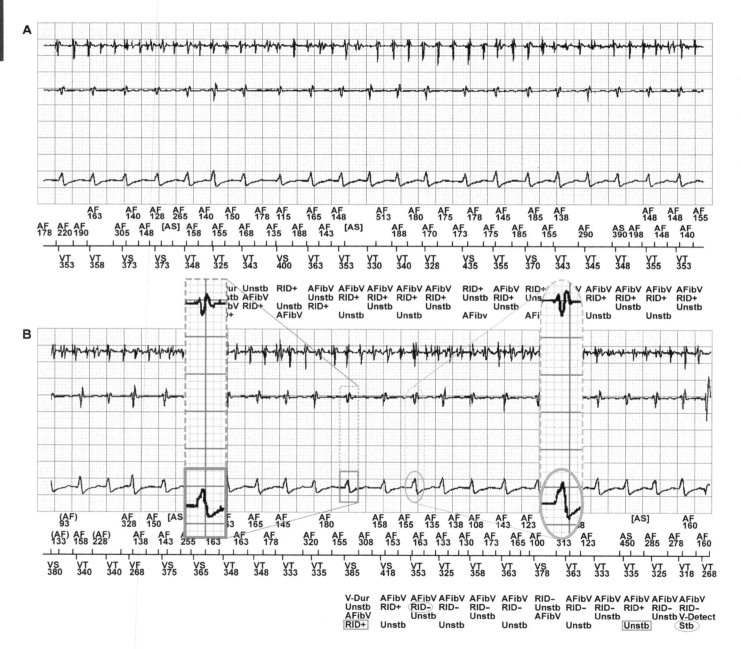

Figure 50.4 Same as Figure 50.1 but with the complex that matches the baseline template (indicating SVT) shown in the square and the mismatched complex shown in the circle. These subtle differences likely reflect minor aberrancy (longitudinal dissociation) during AF.

50

uses both the near-field and far-field EGMs to assess morphology, and changes in either could lead to misclassification (Figures 50.4 and 50.5).

Once the ventricular response during AF exceeds approximately 170 bpm, cycle length variability is diminished and the ability of stability to discriminate SVT from VT diminishes.

Visual examination of the rate and morphology does not suggest ventricular tachycardia, making answer 1 incorrect. Given the multiple

similar episodes, the most likely scenario is that the episode accelerated, thus diminishing variability, and subtle changes in the near-field EGM shifted the alignment of the far-field EGMs, leading to inappropriate detection. The detection occurs in the VT, not the VF, zone, so answer 3 is incorrect. Nonphysiologic signals characteristic of lead fracture are not present, so there is no evidence that lead fracture is present or leads to detection, making answer 4 incorrect.

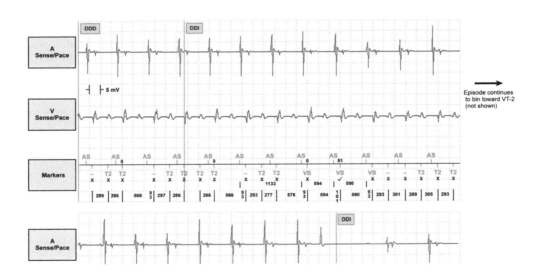

Figure 50.5 Vector timing and correlation to use morphology to distinguish SVT from VT.

Case 51

A patient has a Guidant ICD.

Device settings:
- Mode: DDD
- Pacing rate: 50 to 120 bpm
- Dynamic AV delay: on (150 to 80 ms)
- Dynamic PVARP: on (24 to 250 ms)
- PVARP after PVC: on

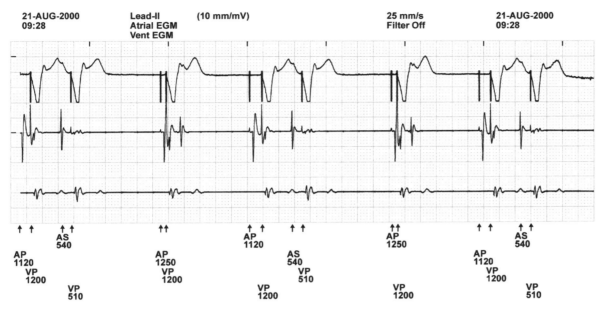

Figure 51.1 From top to bottom: surface ECG lead II, atrial EGM, ventricular near-field EGM, and markers with intervals.

Q: **Which of the following is true regarding the tracing shown in Figure 51.1?**

1. Atrial failure to output is present
2. Atrial failure to capture is present
3. Atrial undersensing is present
4. Inappropriate mode switch

51

2. Atrial failure to capture is present

The tracing demonstrates alternating VV intervals, which lead to variable paced AV intervals (Figure 51.2). The first QRS complex is paced. A sensed atrial complex with coupling interval 540 ms is tracked ("AS" 540 ms, "VP" 510 ms). The short VV interval (510 ms, depicted with horizontal blue arrow) indicates to the device that the heart rate is fast, so that dynamic AV delay shortens the subsequent AV interval, leading to a very short paced A and paced V (asterisk). However, since the second VV interval was longer (horizontal green arrow), the subsequent AV interval is longer. In Figure 50.2, each VV interval (horizontal arrows) and the subsequent AV interval (curved arrows) are shown. Alternations in the VV intervals lead to the variations in AV intervals due to the function of dynamic AV delay, which in Boston Scientific (formerly Guidant) devices measure the preceding VV interval to calculate the following AV interval. Note that none of the atrial pacing spikes (third, fourth, fifth, and sixth complexes) captures the atrium.

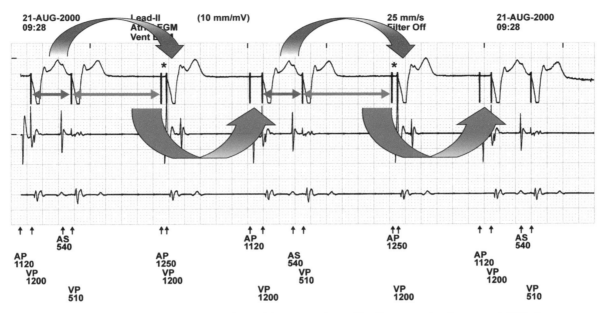

Figure 51.2 Same tracing as Figure 51.1 but with annotations. The first complex is a paced QRS. A premature atrial compex occurs (deflection seen in surface T wave, "AS 540," on atrial channel. The interval is 540 ms (longer than the upper rate limit of 500 ms [120 bpm]), and it is tracked.

51

The role of the AV node in accounting for the alternating intervals is further explained in Figure 51.3. In Figure 50.3, note the first labeled VV interval, with the black horizontal arrow "AVN" to indicate the approximate time interval seen by the AV node as it conducts the paced ventricular complexes retrogradely to the atrium. The paced ventricular complex at the right end of the AVN arrow is conducted retrogradely to the atrium by the AV node (with interval labeled VA). The retrograde A is sensed (AS 540 in triangle) and tracked ("VP" 510, circled). Due to the fact that AVN had just conducted in the anterograde conduction and the VV interval is short, the AV node remains refractory "VP" 510 blocks below the node. Note that at the next complex (at the right end of the purple arrow) the atrium is not captured by the pacing spike. The ventricular paced complex leads to a retrograde A. Since the purple VV interval is longer than the first, black VV interval (by ~80 ms), this retrograde VA time (marked with asterisk) is significantly shorter. This shorter VA interval may reflect decremental AV nodal conduction (the longer the VV interval, the more the AV node recovers and thus the less time needed for retrograde conduction), or may reflect conduction up the fast pathway (with short VA time) as opposed to the slow pathway (long VA time). The retrograde A (asterisk) occurs so early that the atrial channel is still in the blanking period following the "VP" event, so it is not seen and not tracked. Therefore, the next VV interval (black "V-V" arrow) is shorter, leading to a longer retrograde VA interval, and the cycle recurs.

In short, atrial noncapture is present, so that retrograde conduction occurs following paced ventricular complexes, since the atrium remains excitable. Dynamic AV delay and AV node physiology result in alternating intervals. Treatment requires correcting the atrial noncapture, either with reprogramming or lead revision.

Answer 1 is incorrect since there is no evidence of failure of atrial output. Each "AP" is accompanied by a pacing artifact on the EGM, and there are no prolonged intervals without an atrial pacing event. Answer 3 is incorrect, since there is no evidence of atrial undersensing, in that all atrial events seen on the EGM are sensed by the device if it is not functionally refractory. Atrial oversensing is not present, as only the atrial EGMs (associated with a P wave on the surface) are sensed. Answer 4 is incorrect since there is no mode switch event.

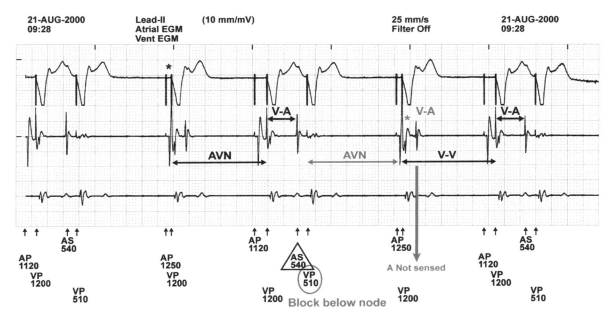

Figure 51.3 Same tracing as Figures 51.1 and 51.2, but with AVN conduction highlighted to explain the alternating intervals.

Case 52

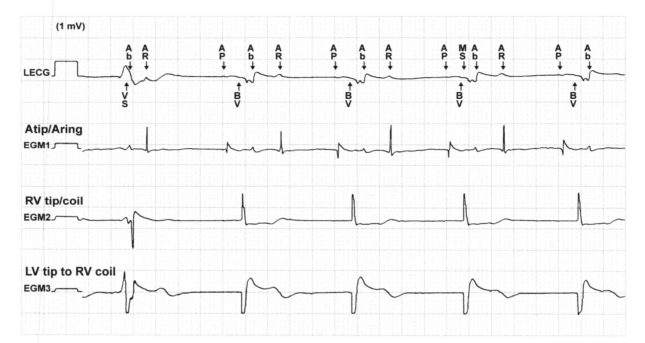

Figure 52.1 Tracing recorded during a routine follow-up visit. From top to bottom: leadless ECG (recorded between an SVC coil and the pulse generator can), the near-field atrial signal (recorded between the atrial tip and atrial ring electrode), right ventricular EGM (RV tip to RV coil), and far-field left ventricular EGM (LV tip to RV coil).

A 61-year-old woman with dilated cardiomyopathy and congestive heart failure received a Medtronic D224TRK CRT pacemaker/defibrillator. During a follow-up visit, the tracing in Figure 52.1 is recorded.

Q: *Which of the following most likely explains what is happening during this tracing?*

1. Double-counting of the QRS complex
2. T-wave oversensing
3. Atrial noncapture
4. Appropriate mode switch

52

3. Atrial noncapture

The patient presents with a tracing that suggests a device problem, in that the number of atrial events recorded by the device on the marker channel exceeds the number of true atrial events seen on the atrial channel (EGM1 Atip/ring). Figure 52.2 is annotated to facilitate review. The first complex (circled) is a PVC. Note that the morphology on a leadless ECG (recorded between SVC coil and can to simulate surface ECG) is different from the subsequent complexes (which are paced, with marker "BV"), and that the first QRS is a sensed event ("VS" marker indicating a ventricular sensed event) without an antecedent atrial event. Additionally, there is far-field R-wave oversensing of the QRS complex itself on the atrial channel (Atip/ring) during the blanking period as indicated by the "Ab" marker (first atrial marker in circled complex). This results since the atrial lead is in the appendage, and records the signal generated by the ventricle (marked with an asterisk on the atrial channel). The second atrial marker is an atrial refractory sensed event ("AR" marker), and results from appropriate sensing of the retrograde P wave on the atrial channel (labeled "Retro P" on the Atip/ring). It is refractory since it occurs soon after the QRS, during the postventricular atrial refractory period (PVARP). Note that QRS itself is seen as a small deflection (asterisk) on the Atip/ring channel that lines up with the "Ab" marker.

In the next complex (down arrow), the AP (atrial paced impulse) does not capture. Note the absence of an atrial deflection on the leadless ECG (top arrow) and stimulus artifact without capture on the Atip/ring channel (lower arrow). Following the atrial pacing artifact a biventricu-lar paced event (BV) is oversensed on the atrial channel ("Ab" marker that aligns with small deflection on Atip/ring [asterisk]). Since atrial pacing did not result in capture, ventricular pacing leads to a retrograde P wave ("AR"). Note that following the third biventricular paced event (starburst/* symbol) the "MS" marker indicates an inappropriate mode switch event.

In summary, atrial noncapture and far-field R-wave oversensing are both present. Markers indicate atrial pacing, far-field R-wave oversensing of ventricular depolarization, and then sensing of the actual retrograde P wave. The multiple atrial events lead to inappropriate mode switch. The problem was corrected by decreasing atrial sensitivity (eliminating far-field R-wave oversensing) and adjusting atrial outputs (eliminating noncapture). No surgery was required.

Answer 2 is incorrect as there is no evidence of oversensing of the T waves. Note that there is retrograde VA Wenchebach, so that with the last complex there is no retrograde atrial conduction through the AV node, and thus no corresponding "retroP" atrial event. The "AR" event is absent in the absence of a retrograde P wave, indicating that it is the P waves and not the T waves that are being sensed on the atrial channel. Answer 4 is incorrect since the mode switch is inappropriate, because there is no atrial tachyarrhythmia present. Mode switch occurs because there is more than one atrial event between QRS complexes, incrementing the mode switch counter. It is inappropriate since those atrial events are actually oversensing events, rather than true atrial events.

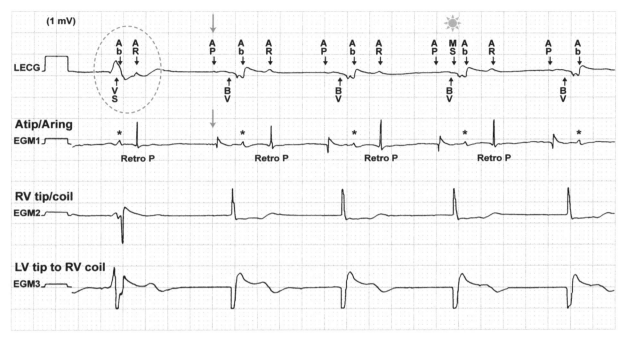

Figure 52.2 Same as Figure 52.1 but annotated.

Case 53

A 63-year-old male with a history of complete AV block, NYHA class III chronic systolic heart failure, and an LV ejection fraction of 25% presented for biventricular ICD upgrade. In February 2002 he presented with complete heart block, and a dual-chamber pacemaker was implanted (Pacemaker: Guidant 1280, atrial lead Guidant 4053, ventricular lead Guidant 4054). In May 2005, due to persistent LV systolic dysfunction, his pacemaker was upgraded to a dual-chamber ICD for primary prevention of sudden cardiac death (ICD: Guidant T125, shock lead Guidant 0185, chronic RV lead used for pace-sense function). In March 2010 the patient was referred to device clinic for symptomatic congestive heart failure and an episode of ventricular tachycardia. Due to persistent LV dysfunction, symptomatic heart failure, and 100% RV pacing from his complete heart block, he underwent an upgrade to a biventricular ICD (CRT-D: Medtronic D224TRK, LV endocardial lead Medtronic 4196). The chronic Guidant 4054 RV lead was again used for pace-sense function and the IS-1 connector of the Guidant 0185 remained capped. Postimplant interrogation and defibrillation testing were unremarkable. The evening following implant the patient complained of light-headedness and an ICD shock occurred at the time of the telemetry tracing shown in Figure 53.1. Interrogation of the episode is shown in Figure 53.2.

53

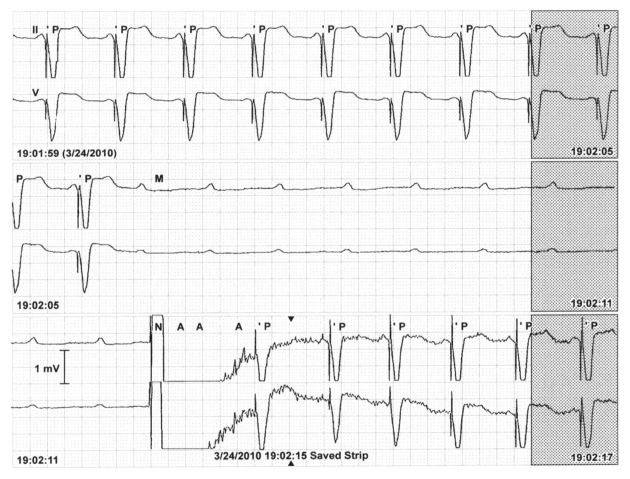

Figure 53.1 Surface telemetry acquired in the hours after device upgrade, associated with dizziness and jolt.

53

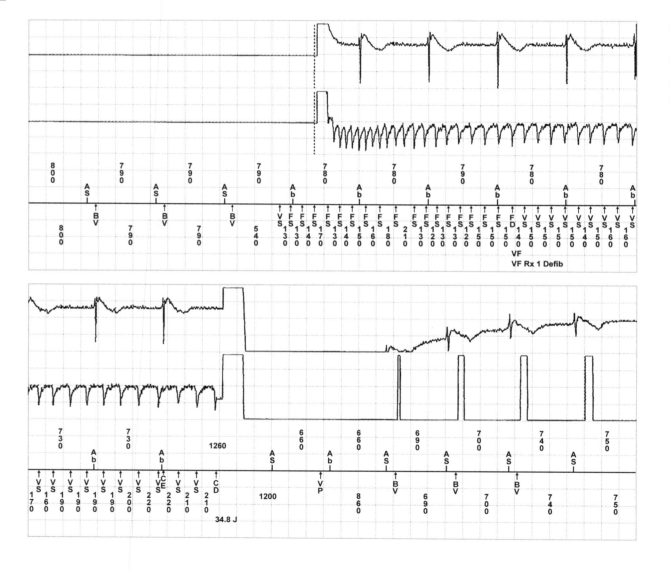

Figure 53.2 Interrogation that corresponds to surface tracing shown in Figure 53.1. From top to bottom are atrial EGM, ventricular EGM, and markers.

What is the most likely cause of the asystole and shock?

1. Crosstalk

2. Electromagnetic interference

3. Loose set screw

4. Air in the header

53

4. Air in the header

Figure 53.1 begins with P-synchronous pacing followed by a period of continued sinus activity, complete heart block, and asystole. The asystole is terminated by a shock artifact, followed by resumption of P-synchronous pacing. This clearly indicates oversensing on the ventricular channel that inhibits pacing output, and that occurs at a high enough frequency to result in inappropriate VT/VF detection. Common causes of early postoperative ventricular oversensing include a loose set screw and myopotential oversensing. Myopotential oversensing occurs more commonly with integrated bipolar leads in which sensing occurs between a tip electrode and distal coil (larger electrodes with greater separation lead to a larger "antenna") than with true bipolar sensing between a distal helix and ring electrode. In this case, a separate pace-sense lead was present (true bipolar). Other possibilities can include contact of the sensing electrode with an abandoned lead fragment or uncapped lead (resulting in make-break noise), air in the header, and rarely (in a recently implanted lead), fracture. Crosstalk occurs when atrial *pacing* is oversensed on the ventricular channel. Crosstalk can lead to pacing inhibition, but not VT/VF detection. In this tracing, atrial pacing is not present, so crosstalk is not present (therefore answer 1 incorrect). EMI, answer 2, is not suggested by the surface tracing, which is noise-free. If EMI were present, intracardiac EGMs would show high-frequency noise that is independent of the cardiac cycle present on both the atrial and ventricular channels.

The intracardiac tracing (Figure 53.2) is diagnostic of air in the header. If minor damage to the header seal plug prevents complete closure after the torque wrench is removed, body fluid may enter into the header via the defect, forming an accessory sensing pathway that competes with normal sensing (Guidant Corporation. Preventing and detecting oversensing due to damaged, torn or missing seal plugs. Guidant Product Update Number 35, November 2003). While sensing is typically not disrupted, if there is air in the header, as the air escapes through the damaged seal plug it displaces fluid, transiently alters the impedance, and leads to nonphysiologic noise signals that can be sensed by the ICD. This form of oversensing subsides after the entrapped air has escaped from the header, and is limited to hours to 1 to 2 days following implant. One treatment option is to program the device to DOO with therapies off and observe for 24 to 48 hours. Another example of noise due to air in the header is shown in Figure 53.3. An image of a damaged seal plug is shown in Figure 53.4.

A loose set screw, answer 3, can mimic this condition. A "typical" tracing from a patient with a loose set screw is shown in Figure 53.5. It is characterized by high-frequency saturated EGMs and not the lower-frequency, more self-similar, regular EGMs seen in this tracing.

53

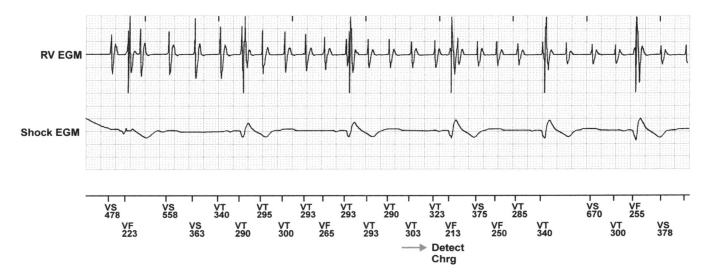

Figure 53.3 Pseudo-VT due to air in the header. From top to bottom are shown the near-field, far-field, and marker channels. Note that on the near-field channel there are multiple signals not present on the far-field channel, due to air escaping the header. The larger, actual sinus rhythm near-field EGMs are clearly seen independent of the artifacts. From Cheung JW, Iwai S, Lerman B, Mittal, S. Shock-induced ventricular oversensing due to seal plug damage: a potential mechanism of inappropriate device therapies in implantable cardioverter-defibrillators. *Heart Rhythm* 2005; 2:1371-1375. Used with permission.

53

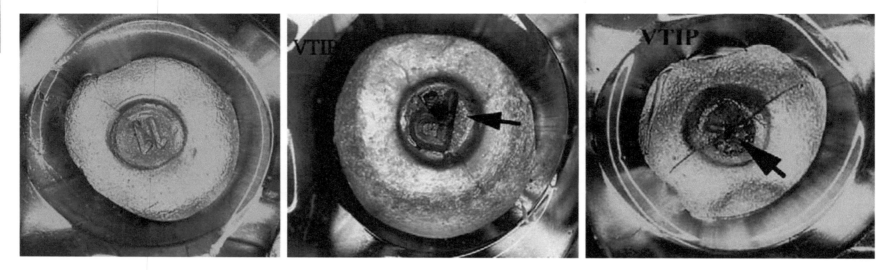

Figure 53.4 Close-up image of seal plug damaged by wrench (see arrows). From Lee BP, Wood MA, Ellenbogen KA. Oversensing in a newly implanted dual-chamber implantable cardioverter defibrilator: what is the mechanism? *Heart Rhythm Journal* 2005: 782-783. Used with permission.

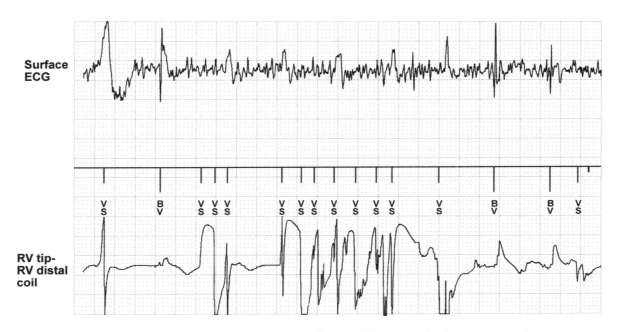

Figure 53.5 Noise due to a loose set screw (from a different patient). From top to bottom are shown surface ECG, markers, and RV tip to RV distal coil EGM. During provocative maneuvers, high-frequency, saturated EGMs that are typical of loose set screw (or lead fracture) are recorded on the RV tip-RV distal coil EGM. There is noise on the surface ECG due to mechanical motion associated with provocative maneuvers.

Case 54

A 67-year-old man undergoes implantation of a Medtronic Concerto II CRT-D defibrillator on LV 4196, RV 6945, and RA 4096 leads. At implant, the P wave measures 3.6 mV, and the R wave measures 8 mV. On postoperative day 1, the device interrogation shown in Figure 54.1 is obtained. Thresholds and impedances are all within normal limits, and similar to implant values. A chest x-ray is unremarkable (Figure 54.2) and upon careful inspection shows no radiographic evidence of system malfunction.

Device: **Concerto II CRT-D D294TRK**
Serial Number: **PZU601715S**

9995 Software Version 7.1
Copyright © Medtronic, Inc. 2006

Sensing Test Report

Sensing Test

	Test Value	Permanent
Mode	DDI	DDI
AV Delay	250 ms	350 ms
Lower Rate	40 bpm	40 bpm

Last Sensing Measurement

27-Feb-2010

P-Wave Amplitude	3.6 mV
R-Wave Amplitude	1.8 mV

Sense Polarity

P-Wave	Bipolar
R-Wave	Bipolar

Figure 54.1 Device interrogation the morning after implant.

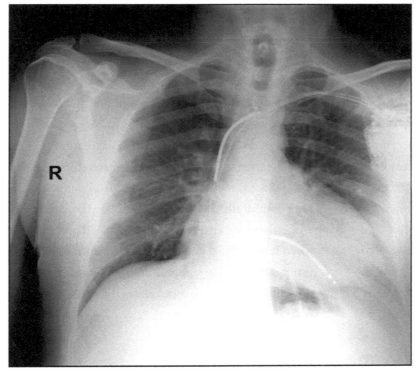

Figure 54.2 Chest x-ray of the patient.

$Q_{:}$ **Based on this information, what is your next best step?**

1. Routine follow-up
2. Reprogram the sensing pathway
3. Increase ventricular sensitivity
4. Decrease ventricular sensitivity

54

2. Reprogram the sensing pathway

The sensing test report indicates that the R-wave amplitude is 1.8 mV, which is a striking decrease compared to the implant values. A small R wave can lead to several clinical problems, the most concerning of which is undersensing of VF. While the correlation between the sinus rhythm R wave and the EGM amplitude during VF is poor, the smallest VF to R wave ratio is typically one-third to one-half. In clinical practice, an R wave at least 5 to 7 mV has been used to ensure acceptable sensing of VF. Undersensing during sinus rhythm in an ICD is uncommon, since dynamic sensing capable of recording signals under 1 mV is nominally programmed in all devices.

In addition to undersensing of VF, a small R wave can lead to oversensing. The dynamic sensing in an ICD increases its sensitivity in response to small R waves; this greater sensitivity during a larger propor-tion of the cardiac cycle increases the risk of oversensing. If the ratio of the R wave to T wave becomes smaller, the risk of T-wave oversensing in particular increases.

Potential causes of R-wave diminution include lead dislodgment, perforation, lead maturation/fibrosis, structural lead defect, and loose set screw. In a newly implanted lead, maturation and fracture are not considerations. The x-ray excludes macrodislodgment, although a micro-dislodgment, in which a small tip displacement occurs, is not detected radiographically and is a likely explanation for R-wave diminution. Mi-croperforations are not uncommon. Lead perforation requires treatment when intractable pain, recurrent effusions, or electrical dysfunction that is not remedied by reprogramming is present. Loose set screw commonly presents with noise that triggers arrhythmia detection and short interval

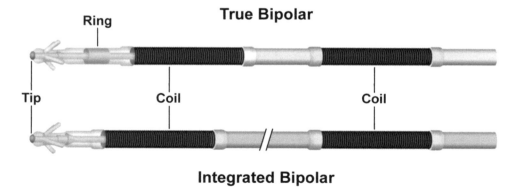

Figure 54.3 True bipolar and integrated bipolar leads. In some ICDs, a true bipolar lead can be programmed to sense between tip and ring or tip and coil.

counters, and episodic impedance elevations. In the present case, microperforation or microdislodgment are the most likely mechanisms.

Of the next steps offered, routine follow-up (answer 1) is not desirable, due to the risk of VF undersensing. Increasing ventricular sensitivity (answer 3) is an option, but the risk of oversensing is increased. Decreasing ventricular sensitivity (answer 4) is contraindicated, as this would further increase the risk of undersensing VF.

The next best step among the options offered is to reprogram the sensing pathway (answer 2). In this device, a true bipolar or integrated bipolar configuration can be programmed. The true bipolar configuration senses between the tip electrode and a proximal ring (Figure 54.3). The integrated configuration, between tip and coil, results in a larger "antenna" since a larger electrode (the coil) is used and the interelectrode distance is increased. The potentially improved sensing comes at the cost of a small increased risk of oversensing, particularly of diaphragmatic myopotentials. In this case, the sensing function was reprogrammed tip to coil, with significant improvement, as shown in Figure 54.4. With each new-generation ICD, the number of sensing pathways for various electrodes continues to increase, providing greater noninvasive reprogramming options, often eliminating the need for surgical intervention. Depending on the clinical situation, other management options include repositioning the lead, placing a new lead with extraction or abandonment of the old lead, or defibrillation threshold testing to confirm adequate sensing of VF with the small R wave.

Device: **Concerto II CRT-D D294TRK**
Serial Number: **PZU601715S**

9995 Software Version 7.1
Copyright © Medtronic, Inc. 2006

Sensing Test Report

Sensing Test

	Test Value	Permanent
Mode	DDI	DDI
AV Delay	250 ms	350 ms
Lower Rate	40 bpm	40 bpm

Last Sensing Measurement

27-Feb-2010		
P-Wave Amplitude	4.4 mV	
R-Wave Amplitude	5.9 mV ←	

Sense Polarity

P-Wave	Bipolar
R-Wave	Tip to Coil ←

Figure 54.4 Interrogation after reprogramming sensing to tip to coil. Note the significant improvement in the R-wave amplitude.

Case 55

A 54-year-old man presents because of a high-frequency device alert tone going off every 4 hours. The patient had a defibrillator implanted 3 years ago for arrhythmogenic RV dysplasia. The device is a single-chamber Medtronic Entrust defibrillator with a Medtronic Fidelis 6949 RV lead programmed as VVIR. A portion of the representative arrhythmia episode is shown in Figure 55.1. The battery and lead measurement report is included in Figure 55.2.

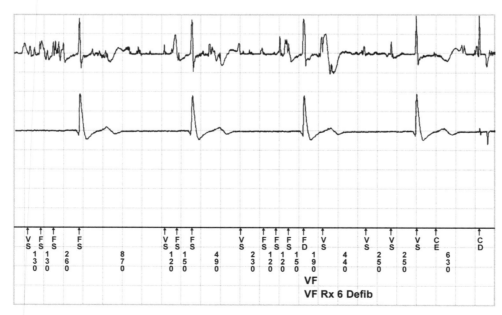

Figure 55.1 Representative arrhythmia episode.

Battery and Lead Measurements Report

Last Interrogation: 25-Nov-2009 11:53:37

Battery Voltage

(ERI=2.61 V)
25-Nov-2009 11:52:10
Voltage   3.06 V

Last Capacitor Formation

20-Jul-2009 12:14:35
Charge Time   9.2 sec
Energy   0.0 - 35 J

Last Charge

25-Nov-2009 04:47:28
Charge Time   1.3 sec
Energy   28 - 35 J

Sensing Integrity Counter

(if >300 counts, check for sensing issues)
Since 13-Nov-2009 19:43:39
Short V-V Intervals   6921

Lead Impedance

25-Nov-2009 11:52:14
RV Pacing   1056 ohm
RV Defib   48 ohm
SVC Defib   58 ohm

Sensing

25-Nov-2009 11:52:04
R-Wave Amplitude   7.2 mV

Figure 55.2 Battery and lead measurements report.

What is the most likely cause for the emission of alert tones and detection of ventricular arrhythmias?

1. Battery failure
2. Electrical reset
3. Ventricular lead fracture
4. A loose set screw in the header

55

3. Ventricular lead fracture

This is a classic example of ventricular oversensing due to lead fracture resulting in spurious detection of ventricular arrhythmias. The audible alert tones signal lead integrity compromise.

An annotated version of a typical arrhythmia episode in Figure 55.3 demonstrates that the device is falsely detecting ventricular fibrillation. On the rhythm strip for this true bipolar lead system, the upper signal is registered from V tip to V ring making it near-field, and the lower signal is registered from can to RV coil (HVB) making it far-field. There are clusters of intermittent, low-amplitude, high-frequency signals that occur at nonphysiologic intervals known as make-break potentials. These are consistent with oversensing of extracardiac signals. The differential diagnosis for extracardiac oversensing is described in Table 55.1.

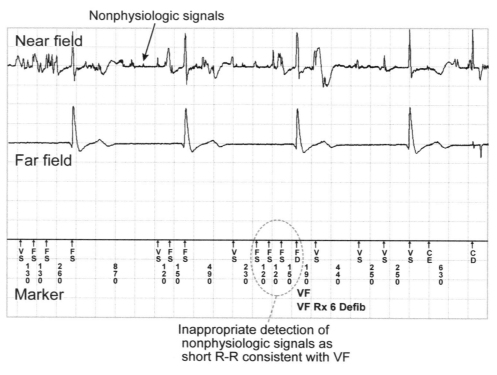

Figure 55.3 Annotated typical arrhythmia episode.

Table 55.1 Extracardiac Sources of Oversensing in Defibrillators

Extracardiac Source	EGM Characteristics
External EMI	Noise on far-field and near-field channels
	History of EMI exposure
	More noticeable with integrated bipolar leads
Skeletal muscle oversensing (pectoral source)	More prominent in far-field when can is part of the sensing circuit
	Resolution when can is removed from the sensing circuit
	May be provoked with isometric exercises
	May result in morphology algorithm error but not inappropriate detection during normal rhythm
Skeletal muscle oversensing (diaphragm source)	More prominent in the near-field
	Potential for inappropriate shocks
	Provoked by deep inspiration/expiration, cough, Valsalva maneuver
Lead fracture or insulation breach	Can effect near-field or far-field depending on the site of fracture
	Lead fracture noise occurs during a small fraction of the cardiac cycle
	Often saturates the amplifier and is very high frequency in content
	May be positional
	Lead impedance may be abnormal (high for a fracture, low for a partial insulation breach, or no change); abnormality may be intermittent
	Potential for inappropriate shock if rate sensing lead is affected
	Chest x-ray may demonstrate fracture, but often does not
Loosened set screw or header-connector problem (including damaged grommet, air in the pocket)	Similar presentation as lead issue, but tends to present acutely
	Lead impedance may be abnormally high
	Chest x-ray may demonstrate a pin coming out from header
	Potential for far-field sensing of pectoral myopotentials
Reversal of defibrillation leads in the header	Large P waves on the shock EGM
	High defibrillation threshold
	Noise (possible pectoral myopotentials) on EGM
Lead-lead interactions	Proximity of 2 leads on chest X-ray
	Normal lead impedance
	More prominent with abandoned or uncapped leads, or extraction fragments in contact with the active lead

Table 55.1 Adapted from Kowalski M, Ellenbogen KA, Wood MA, and Friedman PL. Implantable cardiac defibrillators lead failure or myopotential oversensing? An approach to diagnosis on lead electrogram. *Europace.* 2008;10:914-917.

55

The nonphysiologic and intermittent nature of the signals suggests a lead or connector problem. It is difficult to differentiate the two, except that header-connector problems typically manifest around the time of device implantation or generator change. They rarely manifest years later. Lead fracture in the absence of iatrogenic trauma often has a later course.

Device interrogation was consistent with a Fidelis lead fracture. The sensing integrity counter (SIC) demonstrates 6921 short VV intervals since last interrogation. The SIC is a Medtronic feature based on the concept that very short VV intervals <130 ms (~10 ms higher than the minimum ICD blanking period) rarely represent physiologic events even in ventricular fibrillation. The SIC describes the date and time of the first short VV interval—November 13 (about 1.5 weeks before the interrogation date). It has been shown that abnormal SIC counters alone are a relatively nonspecific finding for lead/connector issues. However, the additional finding of an abnormally high impedance on the RV pacing lead (1056 ohms—increased from 568 ohms at last check) was also consistent with lead/connector issues. Of note, as is typical for some fractures involving the sensing circuit, the impedances of the shock coils were normal. Interestingly, the fracture was not seen by chest x-ray.

The intermittent severity of oversensing in lead fracture (probably due to positioning) and potential for misinterpretation of these problems as intracardiac in origin is illustrated by device interrogation at rest (Figure 55.4). The strip demonstrates ventricular oversensing. In addition to appropriate V sense (Vs) markers corresponding to surface QRS, an inappropriate Vs marker without an associated surface QRS (or ventricular EGM) is also seen. The inappropriate Vs marker tends to occur intermittently at ~200-ms intervals after the peak of the T wave. This may be consistent with the mechanical contraction of the heart.

Answer 1 is incorrect because battery failure would not affect the sensing integrity counter or cause near-field noise. Answer 2 is incorrect because electrical or power on reset typically occurs in the setting of high voltage or magnetic fields. If there was EMI, one would expect continuous electrical signals involving the far-field and an exposure history. Of note, therapies may be turned off for some period in the case of a severe reset condition. Answer 4 is less likely because a loose set screw would likely be observed acutely or subacutely, rather than at 3 years. In this case, the fact that the Fidelis lead is associated with an advisory regarding fracture would also increase your suspicion of a lead problem.

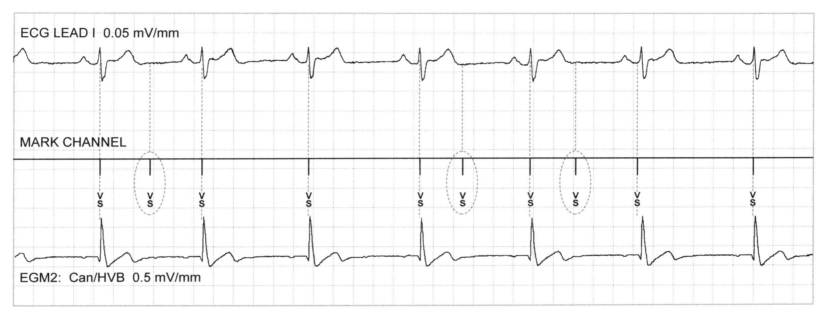

ECG LEAD I 0.05 mV/mm

MARK CHANNEL

EGM2: Can/HVB 0.5 mV/mm

Figure 55.4 Ventricular oversensing.

55

To return to our patient, you make plans for an RV lead revision with a lead fracture, but you are curious that the patient does not report having felt any of the administered shocks. You note that for the last high-voltage therapy, no energy was delivered. For nine of nine attempted shocks, energy delivery ranged from 0.0 to 0.3 J. Programmed VF therapies were for a single 25-J shock (with ATP during charging), followed by up to five 35-J shocks if arrhythmia termination failed. Attempted shock deliveries during the last arrhythmia episode are summarized in Figure 55.5. A rhythm strip demonstrating one such unsuccessful defibrillation episode is shown in Figure 55.6.

Treated VT/VF Episode #100

Episode #100: 25-Nov-2009 04:46:15

Episode Summary		Initial VT/VF Detection Withheld By
Initial Type	VF (spontaneous)	None
Duration	47 min	
V. Max Rate	400 bpm	
V. Median	375 bpm (160 ms)	
Activity at onset	Rest, Sensor = 60 bpm	
Last Therapy	VF Rx6: Defib, Unsuccessful	

Therapies	Delivered	Charge	Ohms	Energy
VF Rx 1 Defib	0.0 J	4.49 sec	<20 ohms	0.0 - 25 J
VF Rx 2 Defib	0.0 J	2.90 sec	<20 ohms	20 - 35 J
VF Rx 3 Defib	0.0 J	1.26 sec	<20 ohms	28 - 35 J
VF Rx 4 Defib	0.0 J	0.92 sec	<20 ohms	30 - 35 J
VF Rx 5 Defib	0.0 J	0.74 sec	<20 ohms	31 - 35 J

Figure 55.5 Attempted shock deliveries during arrhythmia episode.

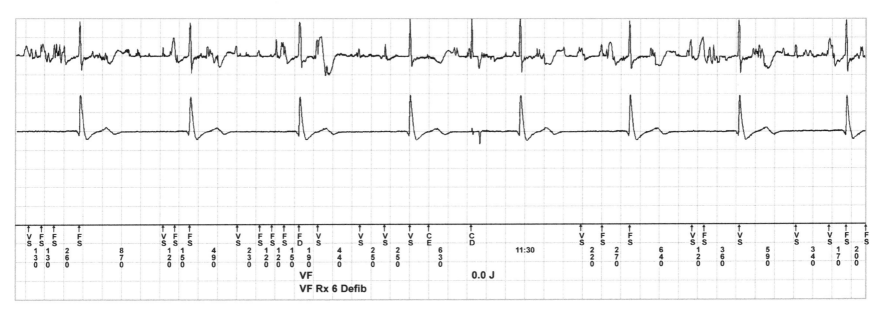

Figure 55.6 Patient's rhythm strip demonstrating an unsuccessful defibrillation episode.

Q: *What is the most likely explanation for the failure to deliver shocks?*

1. Short circuit
2. Open circuit
3. Failure to reconfirm ventricular fibrillation
4. Abnormal sensing due to lead fracture

55

1. Short circuit

Although the device is fully charged, there is negligible energy delivered during shocks. This warrants concern because it is uncommon for lead fractures, even those close to the pulse generator, to disrupt multiple conductors (ie, pace-sense *and* high-energy coils) all at once. It would be presumptuous to assume that replacement of the RV lead alone would be the only necessary course of action, without considering the cause and consequences of the failure to shock.

The description of a very low impedance during attempted shocks (<20 ohms) is consistent with a short circuit. It is likely that short-circuit protection has been triggered. Figure 55.7 illustrates normal energy delivery versus no energy delivery with short-circuit protection. In the scenario of lead failure, an insulation breach can occur resulting in low impedance and a high current. Similar to a home circuit breaker, the defibrillator circuitry monitors current flow during attempted shock delivery. If high currents are registered, a switch is tripped into an off state to prevent further output from damaging the circuit. The delivery energy prior to shutoff is typically less than 3 J, consistent with the 0.0- to 0.3-J energy deliveries seen here. It is important to distinguish this from a failure to charge. In fact, most of the energy remains on the HV capacitors. As the column labeled "Energy" in Figure 55.5 shows, the starting energy after short-circuit protection is a few Joules below the desired shock.

It is controversial how to manage a device in which short-circuit protection is triggered. Some would argue that even though short-circuit

protection is designed to protect the circuitry, inadvertent damage can occur either due to the inciting event (eg, current arcing to can from the site of insulation breach) or due to multiple charge-discharge cycles. It is important therefore to consider whether the generator will be functional with future discharges.

In this case, the patient underwent placement of a new RV lead with sense, shock, and pace capabilities. The dysfunctional lead was capped. The decision was made to replace the pulse generator. The manufacturer analyzed and tested the generator. The inability to deliver therapy was shown to be caused by a faulty capacitor, which was responsible for filtering and holding the supply voltage for the integrated circuit.

Answer 2 is incorrect. Open circuits arise when there is some break or discontinuity in the circuit. An open circuit would demonstrate a high impedance for a high-voltage circuit (>200 ohms). This can arise with lead fracture or loose set screw involving the shock coils. Answer 3 is incorrect because reconfirmation does not occur in this device after the first shock delivery. Confirmation is complete when the markers read FD, or fibrillation detected, on this strip. Charging occurs between FD and CE (charge end). Reconfirmation, which usually occurs between CE and CD (charge delivered) does not occur after the first shock for a given episode. Answer 4 is incorrect because although abnormal oversensing due to lead fracture leads to the detection ventricular fibrillation, it does not directly explain the observation of short circuit.

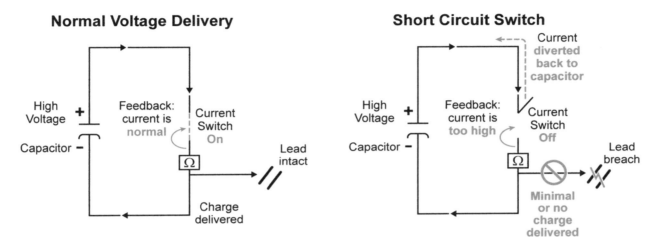

Normal Voltage Delivery

Short Circuit Switch

Figure 55.7 Normal energy delivery versus failed energy delivery with short-circuit protection

Case 56

A 65-year-old man with a history of CRT-D device placement 3 years ago presents to clinic for evaluation of worsened heart failure. You interrogate his Boston Scientific device. You confirm that right ventricular, left ventricular, and biventricular pacing morphologies are as expected on surface EGMs and that lead function is appropriate. Programmed parameters are shown in Figure 56.1. Chest x-ray confirms unchanged lead position. His pacing counters and histograms are shown in Figures 56.2 and 56.3, respectively.

56

Atrial Tachy

Therapy

ATR Mode Switch Details

ATR Mode Switch	On
Trigger Rate	170 bpm
Duration	8 cycles
Entry Count	8 cycles
Exit Count	8 cycles
Fallback	
Mode	DDIR
Time	00:30 mm:ss
ATR/VTR Fallback LRL	60 ppm
Ventricular Rate Regulation	Off
BiV Trigger	On
Maximum Pacing Rate	130 ppm

Atrial Tachy Response

Atrial Flutter Response	Off
PMT Termination	On

Ventricular Regulation

BiV Trigger	Off

Brady/CRT

Normal Settings

Mode	DDDR
Lower Rate Limit	70 ppm
Maximum Tracking Rate	130 ppm
Maximum Sensor Rate	130 ppm
Paced AV Delay	180 - 180 ms
Sensed AV Delay	120 - 120 ms
A-Refractory (PVARP)	240 - 280 ms
RV-Refractory (RVRP)	230 - 250 ms
LV-Refractory (LVRP)	250 ms
Ventricular Pacing Chamber	BiV
LV Offset	0 ms
PVARP after PVC	400 ms
LV Protection Period	400 ms
Blanking	
A-Blank after V-Pace	Smart ms
A-Blank after RV-Sense	Smart ms
RV-Blank after A-Pace	65 ms
LV-Blank after A-Pace	Smart ms
Noise Response	DOO

Figure 56.1 Device's programmed parameters.

56

Date of Interrogation 5 Nov 2010

Brady/CRT Counters	Since Last Reset 17 Sep 2010
Counters	
% A Paced	<1
% RV Paced	9
% LV Paced	91
Intrinsic Promotion	
Rate Hysteresis	
% Successful	0
Atrial Burden	
Episodes by Duration	
<1 minute	0
1 min - <1 hr	0
1 hr - 24 hr	0
24 hr - <48 hr	0
>48 hr	0
Total PACs	0
Ventricular Counters	
Total PVCs	0
Three or More PVCs	0

Figure 56.2 Patient's pacing counters.

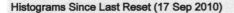

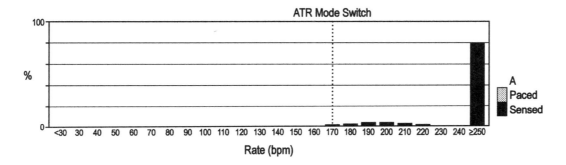

Figure 56.3 Patient's histograms.

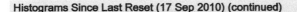

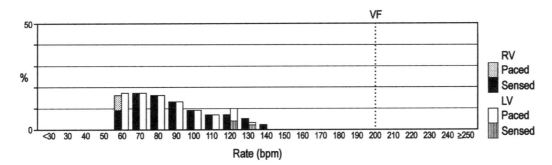

According to the counters and histogram, what percentage of the time is biventricular pacing output occurring?

1. 9%
2. 91%
3. 100%
4. 82%

56

2. 91%

According to pacing counters, this patient receives LV pacing 91% of the time. In devices from this manufacturer, Boston Scientific, LV pacing only occurs within the context of biventricular pacing. An LV paced event may either be in association with an RV paced event or an RV sensed event. If an RV sensed event occurs first, intrinsic activation of the right and left ventricular will follow (assuming biventricular trigger is programmed to off.) When the biventricular trigger feature is programmed on, both right and left ventricles are paced within 10 ms of sensing of an intrinsic, nonrefractory RV depolarization.

While biventricular triggered events represent an attempt at biventricular pacing, it is important to recognize that they do not necessarily represent the same biventricular activation as an untriggered, biventricular paced complex. Rather, in effect they represent a form of "triple site" activation (site of intrinsic depolarization, RV pacing, and LV pacing) with loss of the predetermined offsets. If RV activation is sensed sufficiently early to trigger LV depolarization within an acceptable time frame for biventricular activation to occur, this substitute for optimal resynchronization therapy may still be beneficial. Theoretically, a variety of factors may impact the value of such triggered biventricular pacing relative to untriggered pacing, including (1) the source of ventricular activation, ie, ectopic versus intrinsic conduction; (2) the presence of exit block or slow conduction between a source of ectopy and the RV sensing lead; (3) the relative location of the right and LV leads; and (4) programmed RV-LV pacing offset.

It is also important to take note of 9% of LV sensed events (100%–91%) that do not reflect adequate biventricular therapy. Based on the counters in Figure 56.2, these LV sensed events are probably not attributable to premature ventricular complexes. Rather, this CRT recipient has atrial high rates due to atrial fibrillation. As the histograms indicate, most of the time, this patient has mode switched from DDDR to DDIR due to atrial heart rates greater than the atrial trigger rate for mode switch (170 bpm). For this patient, the biventricular trigger is programmed on only during mode switch (DDIR) but not when he is in DDDR prior to mode switch. That means if an RV sensed event happens at atrial rates above the upper rate limit but before mode switch, a biventricular paced event will not occur in this patient. While there is potential value for maximizing the biventricular trigger during intrinsic conduction of atrial fibrillation with rapid rates, the application of the feature at slower heart rates needs to be balanced with its potential for proarrhythmia. In the setting of frequent left-sided premature ventricular contractions, there is always a chance that triggered events, particularly within the opposite chamber, can create 2 separate wavefronts that may predispose to reentry or other proarrhythmia. Nonetheless, in some individuals, this feature may be considered at rates before mode switch occurs.

Q: *How can you improve the delivery of cardiac resynchronization therapy in this patient?*

1. Leave the patient in DDIR and turn mode switch off
2. Turn Ventricular Rate Regulation off
3. Increase beta blockade
4. Turn biventricular trigger off

56

3. Increase beta blockade

Atrial tachyarrhythmias represent a common scenario in which biventricular pacing may be compromised. When atrial rates are above the upper rate limit but below the rate to trigger mode switch, if AV conduction is robust, rapid, intrinsic ventricular response rates may occur. In this patient, there are 9% of ventricular beats in which the left ventricle is sensed but not actively paced. As the histograms demonstrate, LV pacing initially does not occur when atrial heart rates exceed the maximum tracking rate (130 bpm). Once mode switch to a nontracking mode occurs, the biventricular trigger feature is programmed on and will facilitate LV pacing with all RV sense events up to the maximum pacing rate.

A variety of options can facilitate biventricular pacing. In this patient, an important management consideration would be appropriate rate control of atrial fibrillation. This will facilitate maintenance of heart rates within the upper rate limit and give more opportunities for pacing to occur. This strategy may include titration of beta-blockers or calcium channel blockers, or consideration for atrioventricular nodal ablation in a symptomatic patient. Additional options to optimize cardiac resynchronization in a variety of situations include (1) increasing the upper rate limit to allow LV pacing at higher rates; (2) programming a short AV delay to facilitate biventricular pacing; (3) optimizing sensor settings to facilitate more rapid pacing rate response with activity, in order to compete with intrinsic conduction; and (4) turning on algorithms to reduce R-R variability and increase ventricular pacing during atrial fibrillation such as Ventricular Rate Regulation (Boston Scientific) or Conducted Atrial Fibrillation Response (Medtronic).

Answer 1 is not the best answer. Switching permanently to a nontracking mode has the potential for loss of AV synchrony in patients with sinus rhythm. In a patient such as this who remains in persistent atrial fibrillation, the switch to nontracking mode would likely not help since his device is mode switched most of the time. Answer 2, turning off Ventricular Rate Regulation, is incorrect. Ventricular Rate Regulation was not on in this patient, but it is a programmable option in patients with Boston Scientific devices. When programmed on, ventricular rate regularization functions during the mode switch and is continually active in DDIR and VVIR modes. This algorithm promotes biventricular pacing and reduced ventricular cycle length variability by inserting pacing pulses to smooth out the irregular ventricular events during atrial fibrillation. Answer 3, removing the RV triggering function, is not the best answer. In this device, during mode switch, the trigger function enables RV and LV pacing to occur after an RV sensed event.

56

Case 57

The ECG in Figure 57.1 was obtained in a patient who had a previous dual-chamber pacemaker implanted because of cardiomyopathy. The device was recently upgraded to a defibrillator, and a new ICD lead was placed.

57

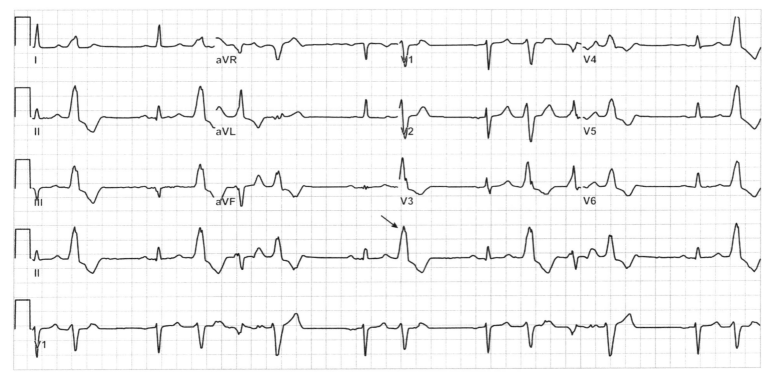

Figure 57.1
Patient's ECG.

Q:

Frequent arrhythmia in the immediate period following a cardiac device lead placement may result from which of the following?

1. Cardiac perforation
2. Mechanical ectopy from a lead
3. Inappropriate programming of the device
4. The presence of endocardial or epicardial leads
5. All of the above

57

5. All of the above

Arrhythmia noted immediately following lead/device placement should suggest proarrhythmia from the cardiac device. The lead itself may produce ventricular or atrial ectopy and nonsustained tachyarrhythmias. The arrhythmias may occur in isolation, or they may represent a complication, such as lead perforation. Occasionally, inappropriate programming (perhaps meant to avoid ventricular pacing) may result in long-short sequences that initiate arrhythmia. Atrial pacing following a sensed PAC falling within a relatively long programmed PVARP may initiate atrial fibrillation. Occasionally an inherent propensity for an arrhythmia such as AVNRT or accessory pathway-mediated tachycardia may be enhanced following device placement due to ectopy or ventricular pacing that initiates the arrhythmia.

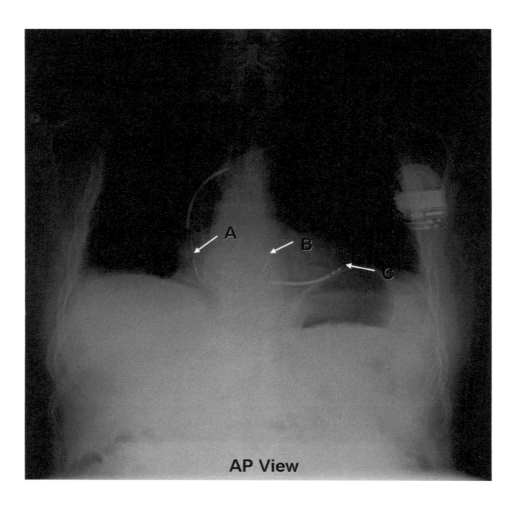

AP View

Figure 57.2 Chest x-ray showing leads.

In Figure 57.1, the wide QRS beats shown by the arrow may result from which of the leads shown in Figure 57.2?

1. A
2. B
3. C
4. None of the above
5. Any of the above

57

2. B

The morphology of the wide QRS complexes often will give an important clue as to whether a postimplant arrhythmia is lead-related or not. The beats shown by the white arrows in Figure 57.2 are characteristic of RV outflow tract ectopy (LBBB inferior axis). Since the outflow tract is in a superior location, PVCs originating there travel toward the inferior leads, and are thus positive in the inferior leads (II, III, aVF). Any event that results in initial activation of the right ventricle (a PVC from the right ventricle, or LBBB) leads to the typical LBBB pattern on the surface ECG. Of the 3 leads shown, A is a right atrial lead, and although atrial ectopy may give rise to wide QRS complexes from bundle branch block, this morphology would not result. Lead B appears to be in the region of the RV outflow tract, and pacing or mechanical ectopy related to this lead may cause the PVCs indicated by the arrow in Figure 57.1. The ICD lead C is not in the outflow tract, and while some of the other morphologies could potentially have resulted from this lead placement, the outflow tract-type PVCs would not occur.

57

The ICD lead marked as C in Figure 57.2 is least likely to be located in which cardiac chamber?

1. RV septum
2. LV free wall
3. Left ventricle via an ASD
4. Right atrium
5. Left ventricle via interventricular perforation

57

4. Right atrium

The AP view of the chest x-ray is not a true anatomic view, given the oblique orientation of the heart in the thorax. As a result, lead positioning using this view can be difficult. By comparing the chest x-ray in this patient with the figure and dissected cardiac specimen shown in Figure 57.3, one can see that the lead may be in a variety of locations, including the RV septum in a counterclockwise rotated heart or in the left ventricle via an ASD, VSD, or perforation. The right atrium is invariably located to the right of the midline and would not be a location compatible with this chest x-ray location.

The lateral view may be helpful in some cases to better define lead location (Figure 57.4). However, this also is not an anatomic view, and several superimposed cardiac chambers may be present in a given location. The arrow points to the ICD lead, which is clearly posteriorly located, sug-

gesting that it is in the left ventricle. In the lateral view, the right ventricle is immediately behind the sternum. The most likely cause of inadvertent LV lead placement is unsuspected placement through an atrial septal defect. The right and left anterior oblique views (RAO and LAO) are true anatomic fluoroscopic views and readily obtained at implant (Figure 57.5).

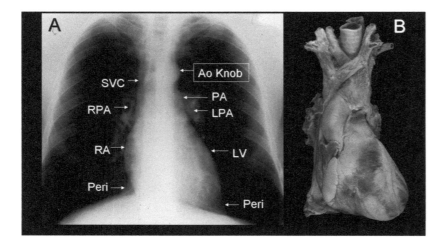

Figure 57.3 Annotated chest x-ray and cardiac specimen. SVC = superior vena cava; Ao = aorta; RPA = right pulmonary artery; PA = pulmonary artery; RA = right atrium; LV = left ventricle; Peri = pericardium.

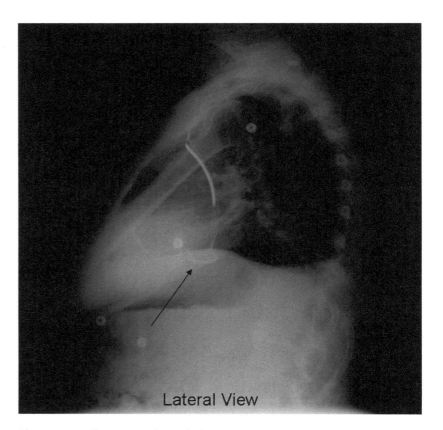

Figure 57.4 Chest x-ray, lateral view.

The LAO view allows immediate identification of lead location in the right or left side of the heart but cannot distinguish between a ventricular or atrial location (in the LAO, we are looking straight at the heart, just as would someone's face, and can tell what is on the patient's right or left with the septum being in the middle). The RAO view is the orthogonal view and distinguishes between anterior and posterior locations. The atria are consistently located posterior to the ventricles, and thus combining information from both views, a relatively precise lead location can be made.

Comparing Figure 57.6 with the anatomic sections shown in Figure 57.5, we note that the ICD lead (black arrow) is on the left side of the body (LAO) and ventricular (RAO). Following the lead, it has coursed from the right atrium toward the left ventricle and appears screwed into the free wall of the left ventricle. Note that although in the RAO view, the pacing lead (yellow arrow) and ICD lead appear to be in the same chamber, in the LAO view the pacing lead is clearly on the right side on the septum relatively anterior in the outflow tract.

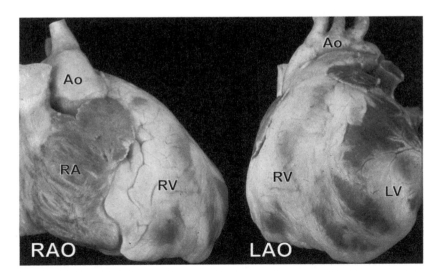

Figure 57.5 Right and left anterior oblique views.

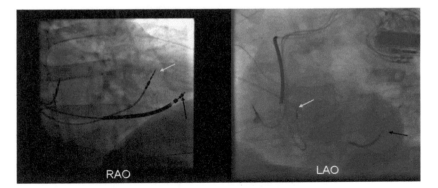

Figure 57.6 X-ray views of right and left anterior oblique views.

57

Several other imaging modalities may be required to ascertain inappropriate lead placement. A transthoracic echocardiogram is shown in Figure 57.7. The posterior location of the ICD lead (white arrow) traversing the mitral valve from left atrium to the left ventricle is seen. The patient had a previous radiofrequency ablation procedure for atrial fibrillation where dual transseptal puncture had been performed. The ICD lead had inadvertently been placed through the septal defect to the left ventricle.

A CT scan from the same patient shows lead placement through the low intra-atrial septum and then to the LV free wall (black arrow) (Figure 57.8). The RV high septal lead is also seen (red arrow).

Figure 57.9 shows the AP and lateral views from another patient who had a single-chamber pacing system implanted several years prior to obtaining this x-ray elsewhere.

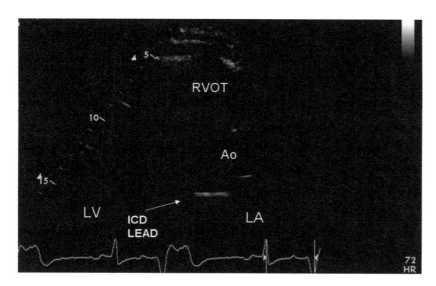

Figure 57.7 Transthoracic echocardiogram. RVOT = right ventricular outflow tract.

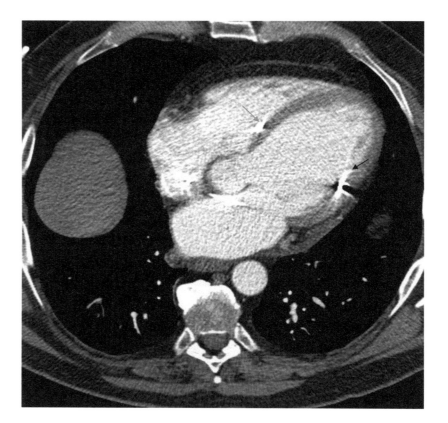

Figure 57.8 CT scan.

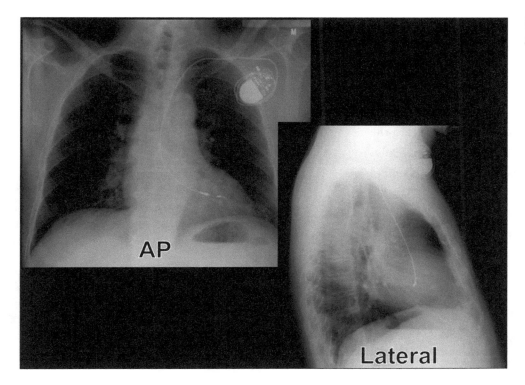

Figure 57.9 Patient's prior x-ray of AP and lateral views.

57

Q: In Figure 57.9, where is this lead likely to be located?

1. Right atrium
2. Left atrium
3. Right ventricle
4. Left ventricle
5. None of the above

57

4. Left ventricle

The lateral view shows the lead is in the posterior ventricle (left ventricle) and the AP view also suggests a leftward location. Unlike the previous example, however, note the course of the lead relatively high with respect to the clavicle and coursing through the midline of the cardiac silhouette, suggesting subclavian arterial puncture and inadvertent lead placement through the arterial system retrograde through the aorta into the left ventricle. Although endovascular LV pacing is occasionally resorted to, it is generally considered to be of prohibitive risk for thromboembolism, even with anticoagulation.

A transesophageal echocardiogram was done and shows the pacemaker lead crossing the aortic valve and being inserted into the left ventricle (Figure 57.10).

In Figure 57.11, note the central location of the aorta (Ao) compared to the pulmonary trunk (PT) and SVC and thus in the chest radiograph, one can usually readily deduce aortic placement versus SVC/RA placement of the lead.

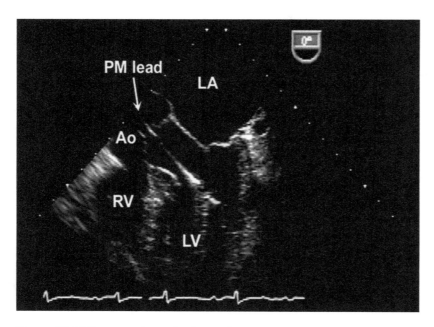

Figure 57.10 Transesophageal echocardiogram.

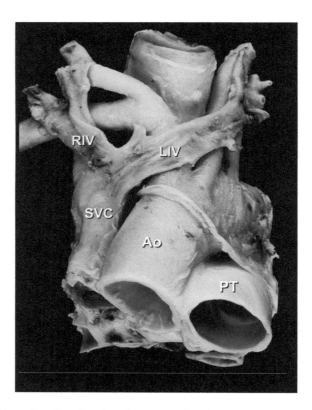

Figure 57.11 Section showing the anatomic relationships of the great arteries and the SVC. Note the central location of the aorta (Ao). SVC = superior vena cava; RIV = right inominate vein; LIV = left inominate vein; PT = pulmonary trunk.

 *The patient's presenting symptom is exertional dyspnea and fatigue, particularly at peak exercise. Given the details of the ventricular high-rate episodes, lead function, and chest radiographs, what is the least likely cause of the patient's symptoms?*

1. Ventricular tachycardia

2. Oversensing on the ventricular lead

3. Atrial fibrillation

4. Loss of atrial ventricular synchrony

58

3. Atrial fibrillation

Based on the high-rate episodes (that show more ventricular events than atrial events, although the atrial lead is dislodged) and the knowledge of relatively poor AV conduction, atrial fibrillation with rapid ventricular rates, while still possible, is the least likely of the given options.

The ideal tool for evaluation of patients with exertional dyspnea and implanted cardiac devices is the stress test.

Figure 58.5 shows the 12-lead ECG obtained during peak stress. Note the appearance of Wenckebach periodicity and suggestion of failure of ventricular output likely from oversensing, which allows the pauses. Given the nonfunctional atrial lead, atrioventricular dyssynchrony is likely also playing a role in the exertional symptoms. Because of the need to exclude ventricular tachycardia, an EP study was performed.

Figure 58.6 shows the AP and lateral projections of catheter placement and lead position at the time of EP study. Note the relatively low and annular position of the atrial lead and the posterior and annular position of the ventricular lead. A mapping/ablation catheter is placed to define the right annulus. Given the possibilities of double-counting and oversensing on the ventricular lead, intraoperative diagnostics were performed at the time of atrial lead repositioning.

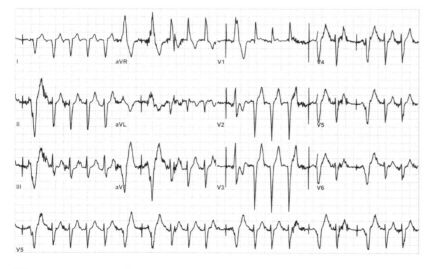

Figure 58.5 Patient's 12-lead ECG.

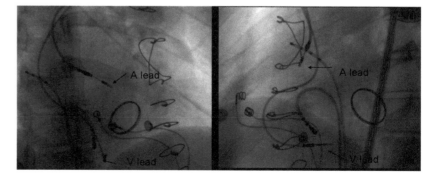

Figure 58.6 AP and lateral projections of catheter placement and lead position.

While we clearly note the obvious problems with the atrial lead, including failure to capture and oversensing, note the normally functioning ventricular lead. There is clear evidence of oversensing in the ventricle, primarily during atrial pacing. The oversensing appears to be related to the atrial paced output near the annulus. Note that AP events are sensed on the atrial channel (Figure 58.7, arrows) at times of absent atrial or ventricular capture on the surface lead. This suggests these events are not oversensing of atrial depolarization (P-wave oversensing) but rather oversensing of the atrial pacing stimulus itself. The absence of QRS complexes at the time of the ventricular oversensing indicated by the arrows confirms that this is true oversensing rather than atrial-lead-induced ventricular ectopy.

In Figure 58.8 we see one instance of oversensing in the V following an atrial paced event with capture (intermittent capture was present). However, at other times, toward the end of the tracing, there is no evidence of atrial capture, but oversensed ventricular events are clearly

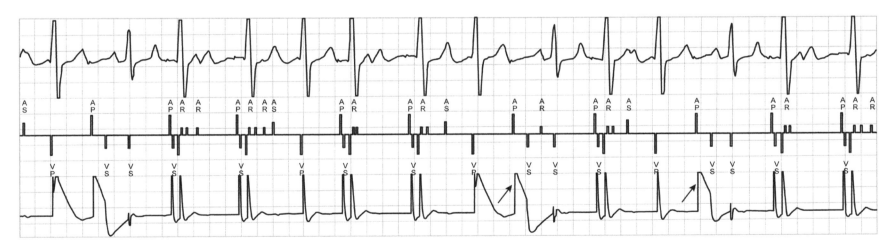

Figure 58.7 AP events sensed on the atrial channel.

58

seen. The distinction between P-wave oversensing and oversensing primarily of the atrial pulse output is important since, if P-wave oversensing is noted, the ventricular lead should be repositioned. However, if the atrial pace stimulus from the dislodged lead is oversensed, then atrial lead revision alone may be sufficient.

Figures 58.9 and 58.10 represent the AP and lateral radiographs following atrial lead revision. The atrial lead has been placed more laterally and farther from the annulus.

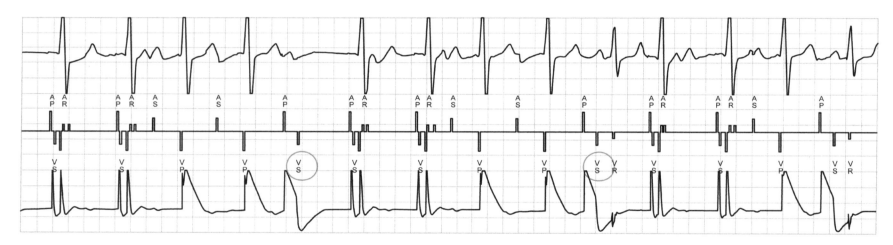

Figure 58.8 One instance of oversensing.

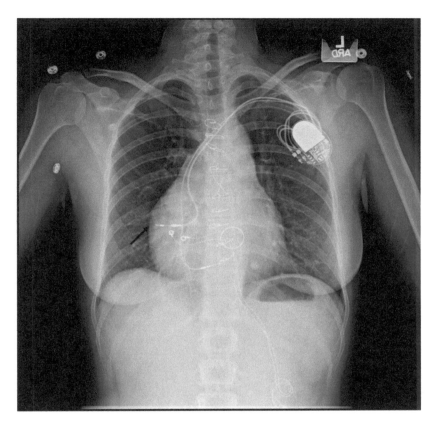

Figure 58.9 AP view.

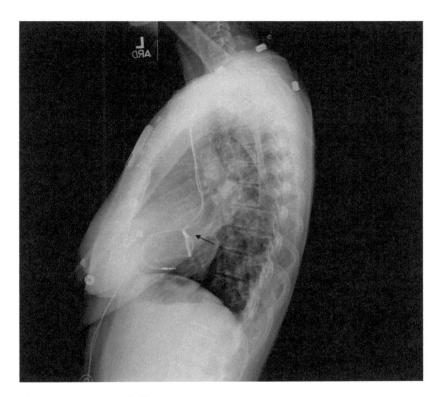

Figure 58.10 Lateral view.

58

Figure 58.11 shows intraoperative diagnostics. With atrial pacing at maximal output and with deep respiratory maneuvers, there is no longer evidence of far-field sensing on the ventricular channel. The patient has done well with no further symptoms at peak exercise and no ventricular high-rate episodes.

Figure 58.12 is the 12-lead ECG obtained when pacing from the ventricular lead (see Figures 58.9 and 58.10 for ventricular lead position). Why is there a prominent R wave (RBBB morphology) with ventricular pacing at this site? Although LV pacing consistently produces an RBBB morphology, there are several RV locations that may do the same. Lead V_1 is an anterior right chest lead. Thus, very apical leftward positions

in the right ventricle and RV outflow tract positions near the pulmonic valve may all have a vector of RV activation toward lead V_1, producing an R wave. In this instance, the patient had congenitally corrected transposition of the great vessels. The right-sided ventricle is morphologically the left ventricle. The lead is positioned posteriorly. Thus, the relatively thick morphological left ventricle is activated from this posterior pacing site toward the anterior/chest location of V_1, producing a significant R wave. When patients present with ventricular high-rate episodes and/or exercise-related symptoms, a combination of an exercise EGM to reproduce symptoms and ECG findings, and targeted intraoperative diagnostics may help clarify the true cause of symptoms and recorded events.

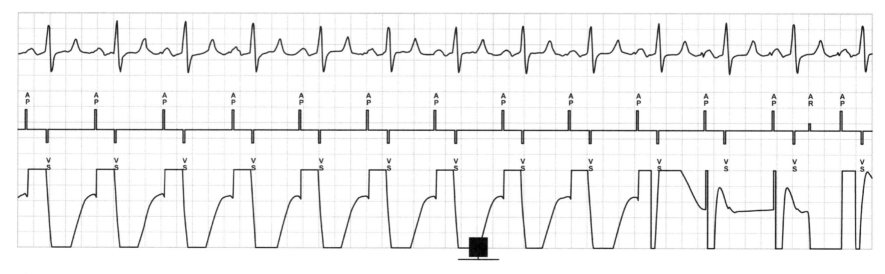

Figure 58.11 Intraoperative diagnostics.

58

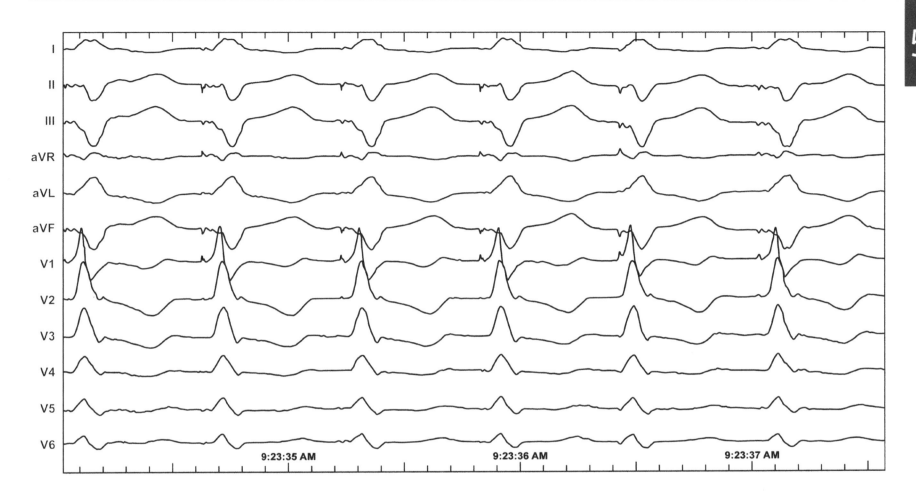

Figure 58.12 Patient's 12-lead ECG.

Case 59

The tracing in Figure 59.1 is obtained from a patient with ischemic cardiomyopathy and a dual-chamber ICD who presents with syncope and ICD shock.

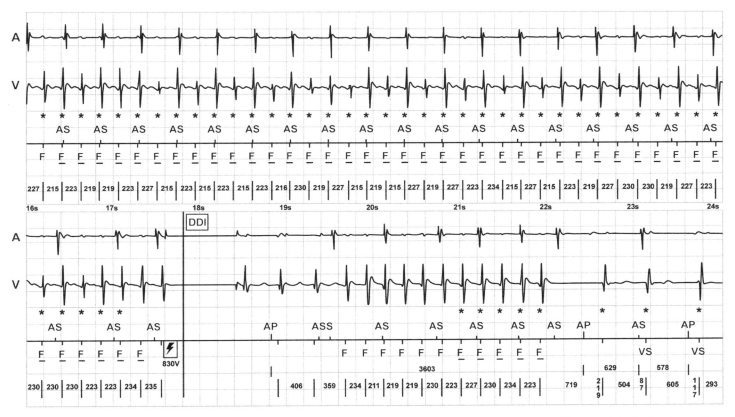

Figure 59.1 Patient's tracing.

Q:

Which of the following statements describes the etiology and appropriateness of shock delivery seen in this tracing?

1. Sensing of atrial events on the ventricular channel leading to inappropriate shock
2. T-wave oversensing leading to inappropriate shock
3. Supraventricular tachycardia leading to inappropriate shock
4. Ventricular tachycardia/fibrillation leading to appropriate shock

59

4. Ventricular tachycardia/fibrillation leading to appropriate shock

The tracing, annotated in Figure 59.2, shows ventricular EGMs occurring at a faster rate than the atrial EGMs (V > A) as well as ventriculoatrial dissociation.

Rarely, supraventricular arrhythmias may present with ventricular rates faster than the atrial rates. Unusual forms of AV node reentry, nodal fascicular tachycardia, and junctional tachycardia are very infrequently seen examples. These discriminations are typically made clinically or in the electrophysiology laboratory.

Answer 1 is incorrect. Far-field sensing of P waves on the ventricular channel may be considered since the ventricular EGM morphology appears to alternate (asterisks in Figure 59.2). However, the variation does not correlate with atrial EGMs. Rather, the variation in near-field, bipolar ventricular EGMs represents a commonly seen phenomenon on

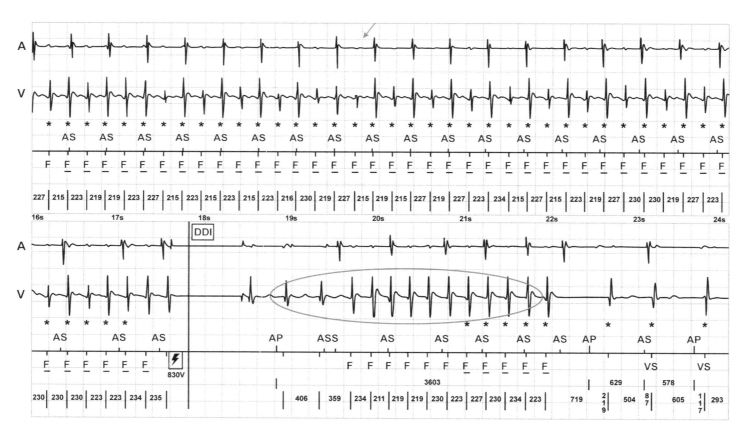

Figure 59.2 Annotated tracing.

intracardiac device tracings despite a monomorphic appearance on the surface EGM. Of note, there is far-field sensing of ventricular depolarization on the atrial channel (red arrow in Figure 59.2). This phenomenon does not affect the ICD sensing of ventricular arrhythmia.

Answers 2 and 3, oversensing of T waves or supraventricular tachycardia leading to inappropriate shocks, are also incorrect. Figure 59.3 nicely illustrates how both can occur at once. In the figure, the patient has a regular atrial tachycardia with variable cycle length. Inappropriate detection of ventricular fibrillation results from counting of ventricular repolarization signals (local T waves) seen on the near-field ventricular (NVF) EGM (arrow) in combination high V counts due to a supraventricular tachycardia.

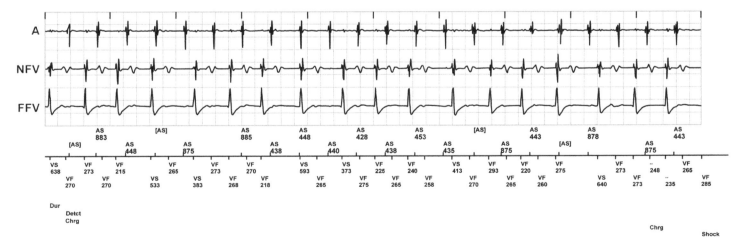

Figure 59.3 Inappropriate detection of T waves during an atrial tachycardia.

59

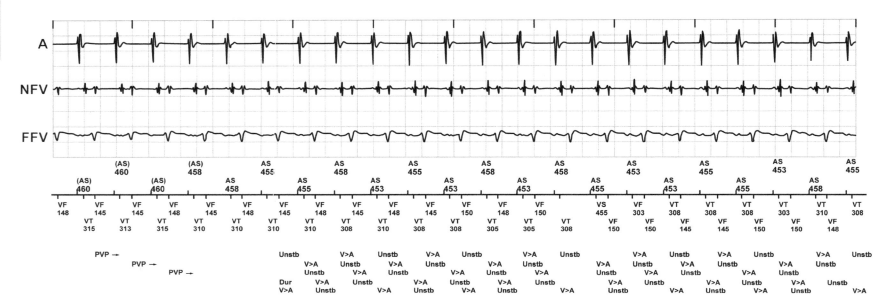

Figure 59.4 Patient's tracing.

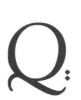

The tracing in Figure 59.4 was obtained from a patient with a dual-chamber defibrillator. Which of the following statements best explains your observations?

1. There is far-field T-wave oversensing
2. Atrial fibrillation leads to shock delivery
3. The defibrillator lead is likely near the tricuspid annulus
4. There is R-wave double-counting

59

3. The defibrillator lead is likely near the tricuspid annulus

This case illustrates the withholding of defibrillator therapy in the setting of crosstalk on the ventricular lead. Because the lead is near the annulus, both atrial and ventricular signals are sensed by the ventricular lead, leading to double counting.

In the annotated Figure 59.5, there are 2 near-field ventricular EGMs for every atrial or far-field ventricular EGM. Answers 1 and 4 are incorrect because the deflection in question bears no particular relationship to either the far-field V, which is not wide, or the T wave. This finding is most consistent with crosstalk on the ventricular lead. Crosstalk is the inappropriate sensing of far-field signals from the opposite chamber. It often occurs in the context of atrial pacing or an annular (or too basal) location of the ventricular lead.

Miscounting of atrial for ventricular signals resulted in this patient intermittently having R-R rates that alternate between the ventricular fibrillation zone and ventricular tachycardia. The rhythm does not consistently meet rate criteria for ventricular fibrillation (in which discriminators do not apply), and thus SVT-VT discriminators can be applied during the redetection phase.

59

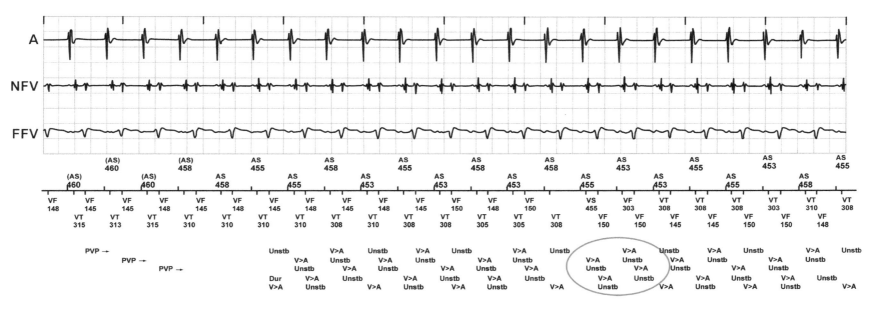

Figure 59.5 Annotated tracing.

59

Depending on device programming, a variety of SVT-VT can result in the *withholding* of ICD therapy. The usual discriminators are rate (actual ventricular rate, and V:A rate), stability (R-R interval variation), and morphology (against a QRS template).

In this case, the therapy is withheld because of irregular/unstable rhythm. This feature (withholding shock for unstable rhythms) is intended to avoid shocks for atrial fibrillation. Inappropriate sensing of atrial signals as ventricular produces a pattern of irregular ventricular signals rather than atrial fibrillation.

The risk of utilizing the stability criteria is mistaking an unstable ventricular tachycardia with R-R irregularity for an irregular SVT (atrial fibrillation). However, typically, unstable rhythms of a ventricular origin will result in classification in the VF zone with no opportunities to withhold therapies. Figure 59.6 demonstrates a tracing from a patient with polymorphic ventricular tachycardia that with rate instability quickly organizes into a fast, regular monomorphic ventricular tachycardia—meeting the criteria for shock delivery.

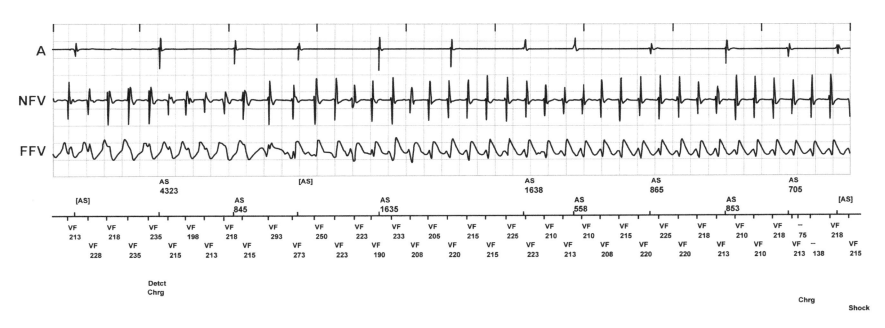

Figure 59.6 Tracing from patient with polymorphic VT.

Q: All of the following defibrillator coil locations may be considered when defibrillation thresholds are high, except for which of the following?

1. Subcutaneous array placement
2. Placing the active can in the abdomen
3. Azygous vein coil placement
4. Epicardial surgical ICD patch placement

59

2. Placing the active can in the abdomen

Answer 2 is the only one that will not improve a defibrillator shock vector. In fact, it has the potentials to worsen it.

Figure 59.7 shows the typical placement of the distal ICD coil and active can in the left infraclavicular region; the shocking vectors between the coil and the can (arrow). Because the left ventricle is posterior to the right ventricle, a large part of the left ventricle is typically excluded from this normal shocking vector. When ICD therapy is ineffective due to high defibrillation thresholds at implant, an alternate shocking vector that incorporates the majority of the LV myocardium into the shock field can be attempted.

In Figure 59.8, an anteroposterior chest radiograph is shown of a patient with acceptable defibrillation thresholds obtained when subcu-

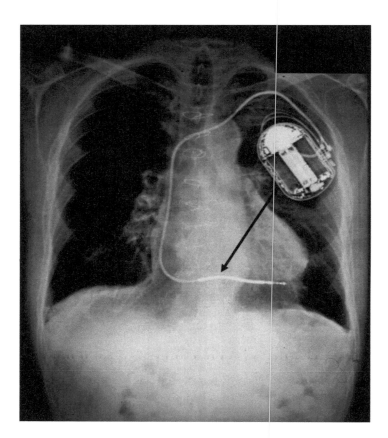

Figure 59.7 Typical placement of distal ICD coil.

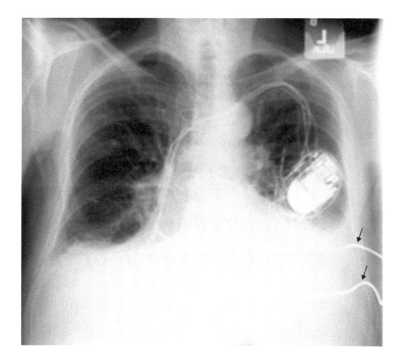

Figure 59.8 Anteroposterior chest radiograph with subcutaneous arrays (arrows).

taneous arrays were placed. The array should be placed as lateral and posterior as possible so as to include the LV myocardium.

Figure 59.9 shows open surgical implantation of ICD patches, clearly encompassing the bulk of the LV myocardium.

Occasionally, the ICD coil can be placed in other endovascular venous structures such as the coronary sinus or the azygous vein. Panel A in Figure 59.10 shows the anatomy of the azygous vein. This vein drains into the superior vena cava and courses from a posterior and leftward course. Thus a coil placed deep within this vein will be located posterior to the heart (left atrium and left ventricle) often improving defibrillation thresholds. Panel B is an intracardiac ultrasonogram of a coil within this vein.

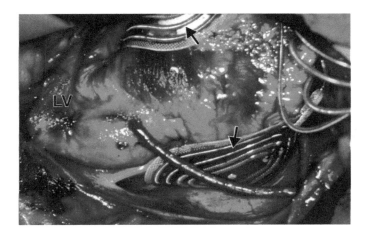

Figure 59.9 ICD patches (arrows).

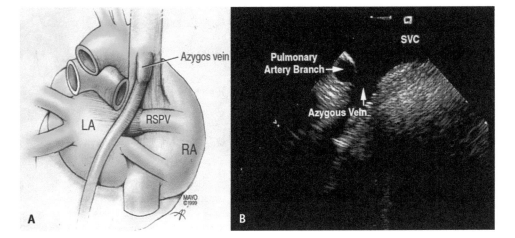

Figure 59.10 Panel A: anatomy of the azygos vein.
Panel B: ultrasonography of coil within this vein.

Case 60

A 52-year-old male with dilated cardiomyopathy and ejection fraction of 27% had a resynchronization device implanted a year ago with initial clinical response. His symptoms gradually worsened because of underlying atrial fibrillation and difficult-to-control ventricular rates that resulted in inhibited biventricular rates. An AV node ablation was performed. Over the last month, he has had progressive dyspnea without obvious clinical cause. RV and LV pacing thresholds were unchanged.

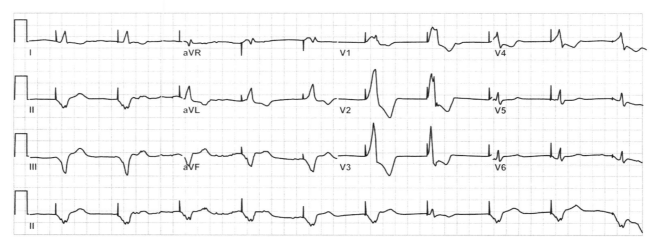

Figure 60.1 Patient's ECG.

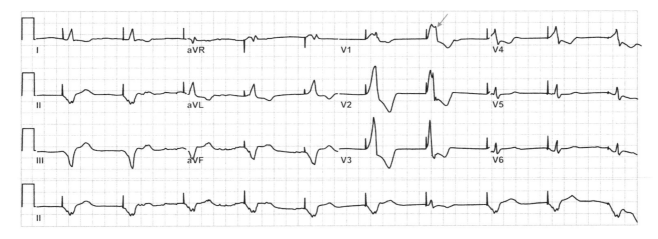

Figure 60.2 Additional ECG showing pseudofused beat.

Based on the ECG in Figure 60.1, which of the following may be contributing to the patient's clinical deterioration?

1. AF with inhibition of biventricular pacing
2. Frequent PVCs
3. Lead dislodgment
4. Suboptimal LV lead location
5. None of the above

60

2. Frequent PVCs

The key finding seen on this and other ECGs was the presence of PVCs. The arrow in Figure 60.2 points to a pseudofused beat with pacing not contributing to ventricular depolarization. The device counters would consider this as a paced event, and one may be misled into believing that 100% pacing is occurring while a significant number of these complexes may be fused or pseudofused. Although AF may also produce fused beats, the patient has had an AV node ablation, and the morphology of the wide-complex beat is not consistent with antegrade conduction through the AV node. On obtaining a Holter monitor and with manual analysis of wide-complex beats, it was determined that up to 20% of the patient's ventricular beats were PVCs, pseudofused beats, or fusion beats.

We can exclude ventricular lead dislodgment based on the information given that LV lead thresholds were unchanged. With regard to LV lead position, the QRS morphology (RBBB, initial isoelectric in lead I, and negative in leads II, III, and aVF) suggests LV posterior or posterolateral placement. However, the prominent R wave in lead I also suggests that programming an LV offset (LV earlier than RV) could be considered. However, the patient's initial clinical response to CRT makes it likely that the lead positioning was reasonable at implant.

There are several mechanisms by which PVCs give rise to suboptimal resynchronization therapy. When PVCs are sensed, the pacemaker will be inhibited, and the PVCs themselves may worsen cardiomyopathy and produce dyssynchrony to the same or a greater extent than expected with single-site ventricular stimulation or conducted rhythm with BBB.

Several device algorithms have been developed (V-sense response, Medtronic; biventricular trigger mode, St. Jude, Boston Scientific) in an effort to maintain resynchronization in the setting of ventricular ectopy or conducted supraventricular rhythms. These features attempt to maintain a semblance of resynchronization by delivering an LV pacing pulse when RV sensed events occur. The efficacy may be limited, however, since much of the ventricle may already be activated by the PVC by the time the event is sensed in the RV. Thus, fusion or pseudofusion results, and for LV PVCs, RV sensing may be a particularly late event, minimizing the benefit of LV pacing at that time.

Other features promote delivery of resynchronization therapy during atrial arrhythmia episodes by increasing the pacing rate as the patient's ventricular response rates increase. While resynchronization may be better promoted, the rapid rates themselves may be counterproductive, mitigating any CRT benefit.

PVCs may be detrimental to effective resynchronization in other ways as well.

Figure 60.3 is from a patient with incessant bigeminal ventricular ectopy. When this condition is frequent, the ectopy itself may produce a type of tachycardia-related cardiomyopathy. The effect on AV synchrony should also not be underestimated. There may be retrograde conduction to the atrium from the ventricular beats, and based on when the PVC is sensed, ventricular pacing may be delayed, safety pacing may occur, or ventricular pacing may occur quite late (circled).

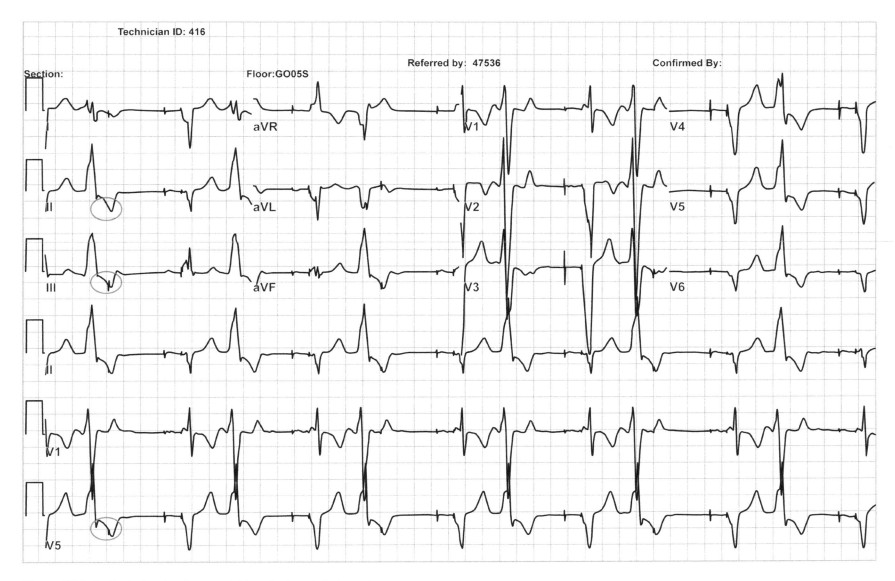

Figure 60.3 Patient showing incessant bigeminal ventricular ectopy.

60

The relationship with atrial pacing is also variable, and nonphysiologically short AV conduction times occur as a result of atrial pacing—PVC and inhibited ventricular pacing (Figure 60.4, circled). In this example, there is alternation between AP and VP (which is delivered as biventricular pacing), and AP and safety pacing (note the double down marker with VS, which indicates safety pacing). Safety pacing is occurring due to PVCs that immediately follow the atrial pacing event. Since the device cannot be certain whether this is crosstalk (sensing of atrial output on the ventricular channel) or a ventricular event, a ventricular pacing pulse is delivered with a shortened AV interval—typically 110 ms.

In CRT devices, safety pacing is delivered only via the RV lead. Thus, in this example, every other complex is resynchronized (AP and VP) and the alternating complexes are PVCs with likely ineffective RV pacing (AP followed by VS with double marker). Note that the small but visible far-field R wave in the atrial EGM indicates the different morphology QRS for each of the pacing types. The clearly visible and nonsaturated ventricular EGM favors the presence of PVCs as opposed to crosstalk. Additionally, since ventricular sensitivity increases over time in defibrillators following each paced beat, the fact that the safety pacing occurs following shorter intervals (VP to VS interval) rather than longer ones

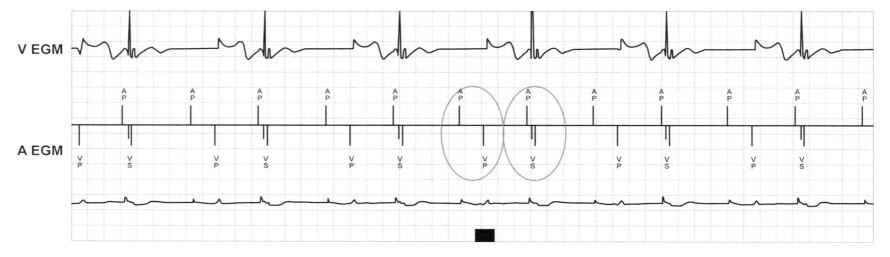

Figure 60.4 PVC and inhibited ventricular pacing.

argues against crosstalk and favors these events as being PVCs that trigger safety pacing.

A single PVC may result not only in inhibition of one resynchronized paced beat but in continuous promotion of intrinsic conduction and continued suppression of biventricular pacing. This results from functional undersensing in the atrium as illustrated in Figure 60.5. With most devices, following a PVC, the PVARP is extended. Either retrograde conduction from the PVC or the next sinus beat may fall in this extended PVARP and will not be tracked. Atrial pacing may then occur, but since the atrium is refractory, it will not capture, and if antegrade conduction through the AV node is present, then the sinus beats falling in the PVARP will conduct to the ventricle (Figure 60.6), and this, in turn, will result in persistent loss of biventricular pacing and continued antegrade conduction of sinus rhythm.

In some cardiac devices (Medtronic—atrial tracking recovery), features are designed to promote AV synchrony even if temporarily lost during a PVC or rapid atrial rhythm by temporarily shortening the PVARP to regain atrial tracking.

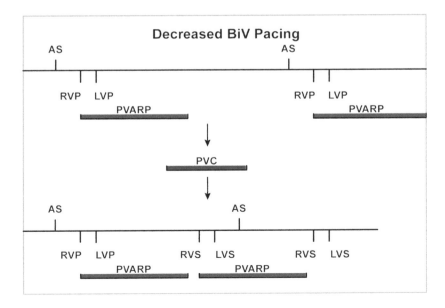

Figure 60.5 Decreased biventricular pacing.

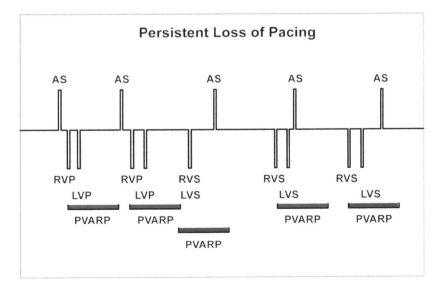

Figure 60.6 Persistent loss of pacing.

60

The ECG in Figure 60.7 shows frequent atrial ectopy. Although atrial ectopy is not generally as symptomatic as PVCs, they also result in several features similarly detrimental to resynchronization. AV synchrony is not maintained in a consistent fashion, as shown in the figure. A premature atrial beat or increase in the sinus rate may also give rise to functional undersensing with antegrade conduction and potential perpetuation of inhibition of biventricular pacing (not shown).

Higher atrial rates, frequent premature atrial and ventricular beats, and the presence of antegrade delayed AV conduction (a long PR interval) all promote this phenomenon and may prevent biventricular

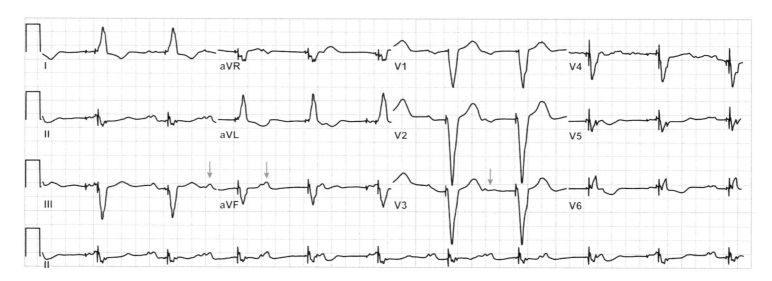

Figure 60.7 ECG showing frequent atrial ectopy.

stimulation, thus lowering the total "dose" of resynchronization (Figure 60.8). The key interval to keep in mind when troubleshooting insufficient biventricular pacing is that the total atrial refractory period (TARP) is the sum of the sensed AV interval and the PVARP. By preventing rapid rates in the atrium (beta-blockers), PVCs and PACs (antiarrhyth-

mic drugs, ablation), and shortening the PVARP when possible (atrial tracking, recovery, turning off PVC PVARP extension) the frequency of biventricular pacing is increased. Conversely, algorithms to terminate pacemaker-mediated tachycardia (PMT) may interrupt CRT delivery by promoting intrinsic rhythms.

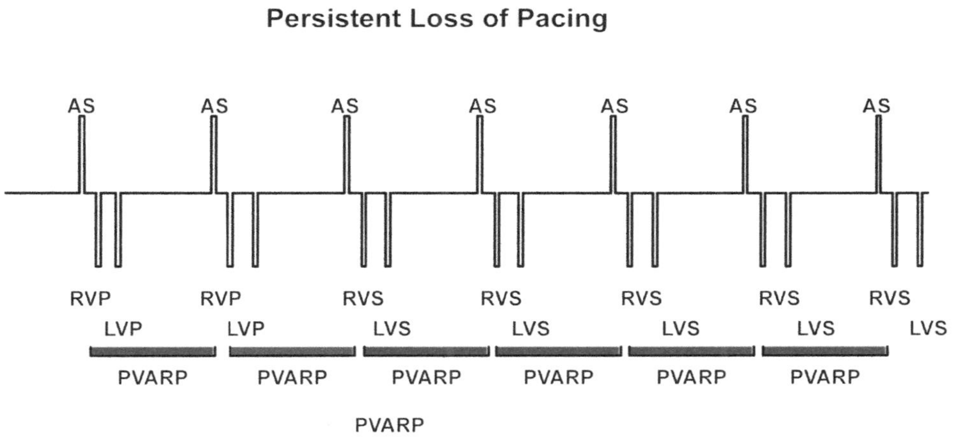

Persistent Loss of Pacing

Figure 60.8 High atrial rate: persistent loss of pacing.

60

Figure 60.9 is an ECG from a patient with a CRT device placed 1 year ago in sinus rhythm.

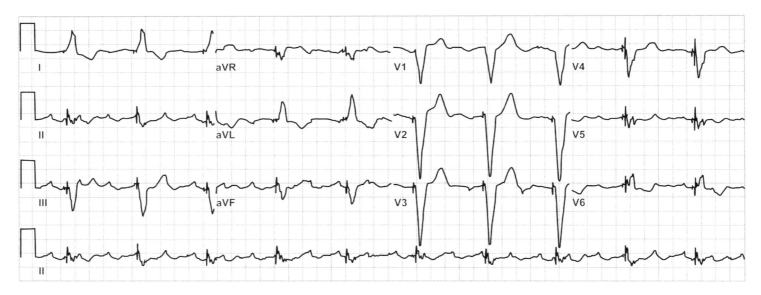

Figure 60.9 Patient's ECG.

In Figure 60.9, what is the most likely cause of abrupt clinical deterioration?

1. Functional undersensing
2. Failure to capture
3. Atrial flutter
4. Frequent PVCs
5. None of the above

60

3. Atrial flutter

Regular atrial flutter waves are shown by arrows in Figure 60.10. The patient's rhythm has changed, and often temporal correlation with clinical deterioration will be evident. Although the same syndrome may occur with AF, in atrial flutter, because of continued organized atrial activity, symptoms are often more pronounced as AV dyssynchrony is caused by poorly timed flutter contractions, as opposed to the complete loss of AV synchrony associated with AF due to the lack of meaningful atrial activity. Thus, with flutter, symptoms may be more pronounced even when ventricular rates are well controlled and CRT therapy is otherwise delivered. This patient had a marked improvement in symptoms with cardioversion and was subsequently treated with radiofrequency ablation. Atrial ATP may also be appropriate in some cases, but at present CRT devices with atrial ATP therapy are not available. In selected patients, use of an ATP device with Y-adapted RV and LV leads may be tried to get both the benefits of maintaining sinus rhythm and CRT when radiofrequency ablation and antiarrhythmic drug therapy fails. However, adapting RV and LV leads in defibrillators is generally avoided due to the significant risk of R-wave double-counting and inappropriate shock.

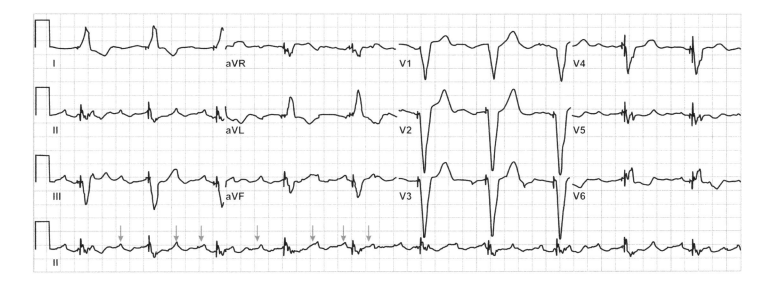

Figure 60.10 Regular atrial flutter waves.

Case 61

The tracings in Figure 61.1 were obtained from a 70-year-old male with a dual-chamber ICD placed for sinus node dysfunction and ischemic cardiomyopathy; the EGMs were recorded during testing.

Device settings:
- Mode: DDDt
- Pacing rate: 85 bpm
- PAV interval: 120 ms
- PVARP: 250 ms
- PVAB: 50 ms
- Atrial sensitivity: 0.4 mV
- Ventricular sensitivity: 2 mV
- Atrial output: 4 V at 0.4 ms
- Ventricular output: 4 V at 0.4 ms

61

Figure 61.1
Patient's EGMs.

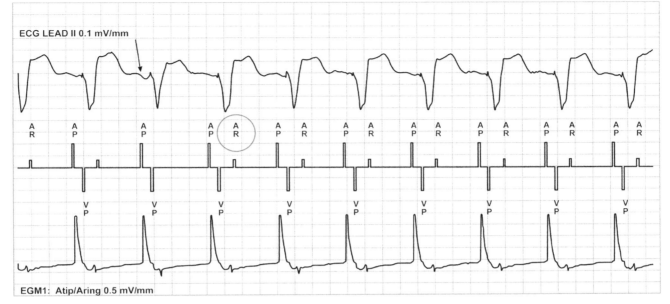

ECG LEAD II 0.1 mV/mm

EGM1: Atip/Aring 0.5 mV/mm

Circled in this tracing are events annotated AR representing atrial events sensed during the PVARP. All of these are true of the AR events except for which of the following?

1. May represent far-field sensing of a ventricular event
2. May represent retrograde ventriculoatrial (VA) conduction
3. May be eliminated or made less frequent by decreasing the atrial sensitivity (making it less sensitive)
4. May be eliminated or made less frequent by extending the PVARP
5. Are of no consequence and can be ignored

61

4. May be eliminated or made less frequent by extending the PVARP

The tracing demonstrates sequential AV pacing followed by a sensed atrial event (AR) in the PVARP. One potential cause is far-field sensing of ventricular depolarization (answer 1). Such events may be of clinical significance in ICD systems since during ventricular tachycardia with retrograde VA conduction 2 "atrial" events would be sensed for every ventricular event on the ventricular channel, thus mimicking a supraventricular tachycardia process and potentially withholding ICD therapy. In the tracings shown, however, the most likely cause is VA conduction from ventricular pacing (answer 2). The arrow points to a beat where a distinct P wave can be seen following the atrial pacing stimulus.

This suggests atrial capture. On that beat, there is no sensed atrial event in the PVARP. In all the subsequent beats, there is no clear evidence of atrial capture, and retrograde VA conduction may thus be allowed and the sensed events in the PVARP detected. One cannot rule out the possibility on this tracing alone that atrial capture occurs in all beats, and the reason for the lack of a far-field ventricular signal on beat number 3 may be a fused PVC with a different ventricular activation sequence. Regardless, extending the PVARP will not change the likelihood of seeing such AR events. Making the atrial channel less sensitive could prevent detection of these atrial events. In certain patients with poorly sensed atrial EGMs, particularly in atrial fibrillation leading to mode switch, one may program the atrial sensitivity to a very sensitive value, thus increasing the likelihood of detecting far-field ventricular depolarization on the atrial channel. In several clinical scenarios with ICDs, CRT devices, and regular pacemakers, such AR events may result in clinically significant sequelae and cannot always be ignored (see next).

Figures 61.2 and 61.3 are from a patient with ischemic cardiomyopathy implanted with an older CRT-D device where the LV and RV leads are Y-adapted to the ventricular port. After an initial response to cardiac resynchronization, he developed worsening heart failure 6 months after implantation. He is 93% ventricular paced.

Device parameters:
- Mode: DDDR
- Pacing rate: 85 bpm
- PAV: 130 ms
- SAV: 160 ms
- PVARP: 320 ms
- PMT response and PVC response: on
- Atrial sensitivity: 0.5 mV; ventricular sensitivity: 2 mV
- Atrial output: 2 V at 0.4 ms, ventricular output: 2.5 V at 0.4 ms
- Measured P wave: 3 mV; R wave: 6 mV

61

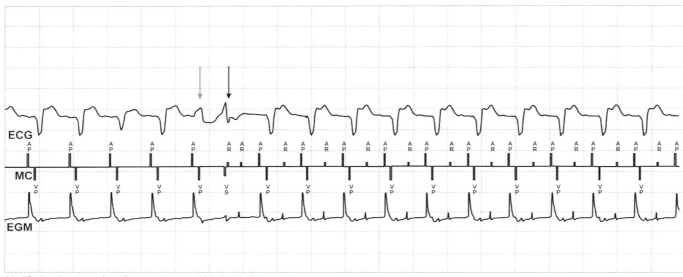

Figure 61.2 Patient's tracing.

Modified and redrawn from figures courtesy of Medtronic, Inc.

61

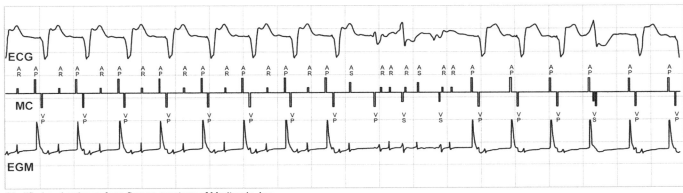

Figure 61.3 Patient's tracing.

Modified and redrawn from figures courtesy of Medtronic, Inc.

Q: *Based on these tracings, what is the most likely cause for the patient's clinical deterioration?*

1. Failure to capture on the LV lead
2. Low percentage of biventricular pacing
3. Ineffective biventricular pacing due to dyssynchronous AV pacing
4. Improper LV lead positioning

61

3. Ineffective biventricular pacing due to dyssynchronous AV pacing

As mentioned, the AR sensed events during the PVARP may represent retrograde atrial activation or far-field sensing of ventricular depolarization.

As demonstrated on the atrial EGMs in Figure 61.4, both the far-field EGMs as well as true retrograde atrial activation can be distinguished. At the beginning of the tracing there is AV sequential pacing. The red arrow is a PVC of one morphology that is timed such that retrograde atrial activation does not occur. A second PVC (black arrow) does result in retrograde atrial activation and creates the first AR event

(circled). Atrial pacing occurs at the programmed interval, but because the atrial tissue is refractory, capture does not occur, thus when ventricular pacing after the programmed PAV occurs, there is no antegrade conduction into the AV node (failure of atrial capture and allows retrograde ventricular activation, VA activation again giving rise to atrial depolarization during the PVARP). Once again, atrial pacing at the programmed rate occurs without the capture, and the situation repeats itself. What is the physiological result of this sequence? The patient essentially has dyssynchronous AV activation with retrograde atrial activation from ventricular pacing and in essence a "pacemaker syndrome"

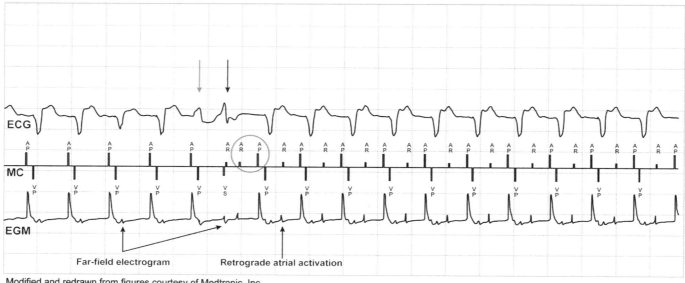

Figure 61.4 Annotated atrial EGMs.

Modified and redrawn from figures courtesy of Medtronic, Inc.

occurring despite a dual-chamber system with normal sensing and capture in both chambers.

The situation is further exacerbated since most devices automatically extend the PVARP after a PVC (PVC response). While this reduces the chance of pacemaker-mediated tachycardia, dyssynchronous AV pacing may be facilitated by the extended PVARP.

In Figure 61.5 we note that a different timed PVC sequence gives rise to earlier retrograde activation, allowing enough time for atrial recovery, and now the paced output captures the atrium, and there is restoration of AV synchronous pacing.

With regard to the other options in the question, there is evidence of appropriate LV capture (answer 1), as well as evidence of a reasonable percentage of ventricular pacing (answer 2), and the initial response to CRT suggests that lead positioning was optimal (answer 4). Frequent ectopy is often the cause for initiating the sequence of dyssynchronous AV pacing.

Frequent PVCs in CRT systems have the potential to reduce effectiveness through frequent fusion and pseudofusion, functional undersensing and loss of ventricular pacing, persistent loss of pacing, AV dyssynchrony, and induction of arrhythmia and PVC-induced cardiomyopathy.

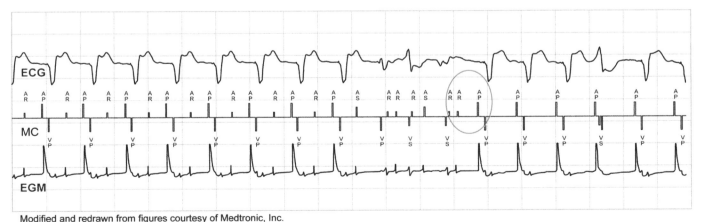

Figure 61.5 Tracing showing earlier retrograde activation.

Modified and redrawn from figures courtesy of Medtronic, Inc.

61

The effect of PVCs on creating a loss of synchronous biventricular pacing is shown in Figure 61.6. Note the PVC (RVS LVS) is associated with PVARP extension and retrograde conduction to the atrium, beginning the cycle of persistent AV dyssynchrony.

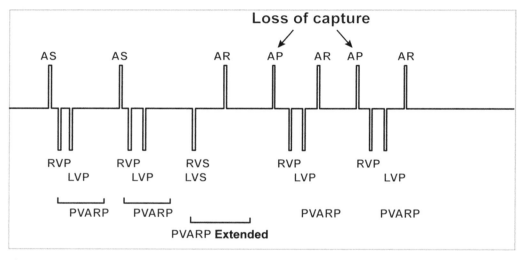

Figure 61.6 Loss of synchronous biventricular pacing.

Which of the following would represent an optimal method in preventing dyssynchronous AV pacing?

1. Shortening VA conduction time
2. Extending the PVARP
3. Decreasing the paced AV interval
4. Increasing the upper tracking rate

61

3. Decreasing the paced AV interval

The crux of solving this problem lies in optimizing the interval between ventricular pacing, retrograde atrial sensing (AR) within the PVARP, and the *next* atrial paced impulse (AP). A sufficiently long interval between the AR and the subsequent AP will allow time for recovery from atrial refractoriness and thus atrial capture, which in turn will prevent retrograde VA activation after ventricular pacing. Since the VP-AP interval cannot be directly programmed, shortening the AP-VP interval will achieve this result. Shortening the PVARP will also get rid of the present problem of AV dissociation, but is likely to predispose pacemaker-mediated tachycardia, especially in a patient such as this with frequent PVCs. Lengthening VA conduction time or blocking VA conduction altogether with an AV nodal blocking agent may also be appropriate in certain cases. Such agents may suppress ventricular ectopy, as well.

In Figure 61.7 the effect of programming a short PAV (100 ms) is shown. In effect, the atrial paced event occurs later (closer to the next ventricular paced beat), thus allowing time for atrial recovery and capture in the atrium. Following this, synchronous AV pacing results. Note that despite shortening the AV interval, AV dissociation continues for a while until a PVC terminates it by further prolonging the AR-AP interval and thus allowing atrial capture.

Figure 61.8 shows the further beneficial effect of reducing the pacing rate. Despite programming the PAV at 100 ms, AV dyssynchronous pacing continued to occur with frequent PVCs. With the PAV remaining at 100 ms, the pacing rate was reduced to 80 bpm. By prolonging the paced cycle length, further time is allowed (nearly 400 ms) for atrial refractoriness to recover, and synchronous AV pacing ensues.

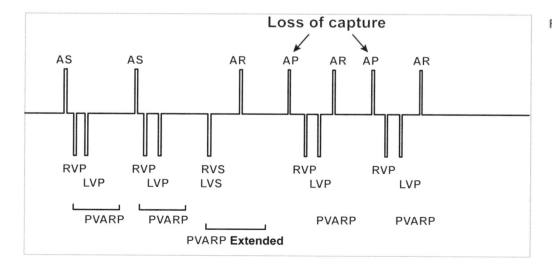

Figure 61.7 Effect of programming a short PAV.

In Figure 61.9 (panel A), we note the effect of simply shortening the PVARP. The PVARP was shortened to 310 ms, and while AV dyssynchronous pacing no longer occurred, given the patient's PVCs, a PVC results in VA conduction, which still just falls in the PVARP. Atrial pacing then occurs without capture. This time, VA conduction is sufficiently long so that the retrograde atrial event is sensed and tracked, giving rise to a short run of pacemaker-mediated tachycardia. This is remedied by increasing the PVARP (panel B) to 340 ms; however, when a PVC occurs, AV pacing ensues.

Patients with frequent PVCs and marked symptoms compatible with pacemaker syndrome should be evaluated for possibly dissociated AV pacing. Appropriate changes in the AV interval or possibly the pacing rate may solve the problem.

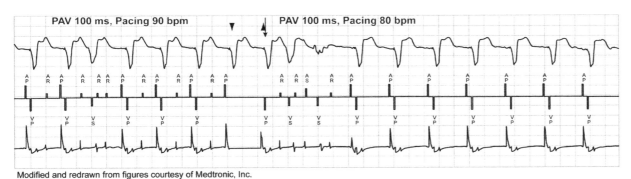

Modified and redrawn from figures courtesy of Medtronic, Inc.

Figure 61.8 Beneficial effect of reducing the pacing rate.

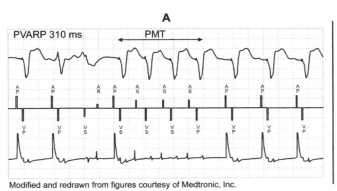

Modified and redrawn from figures courtesy of Medtronic, Inc.

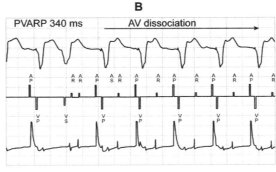

Figure 61.9 Panel A: shortening the PVARP. Panel B: increasing the PVARP.

Case 62

You are called to evaluate an elderly male with atrial fibrillation and ischemic cardiomyopathy noted on telemetry to have varying pacing intervals. He has a Boston Scientific biventricular ICD system in place. The patient is hospitalized for a gastrointestinal illness, and the service is concerned there is device malfunction.

On interrogation of the device, the tracing in Figure 62.1 is obtained.

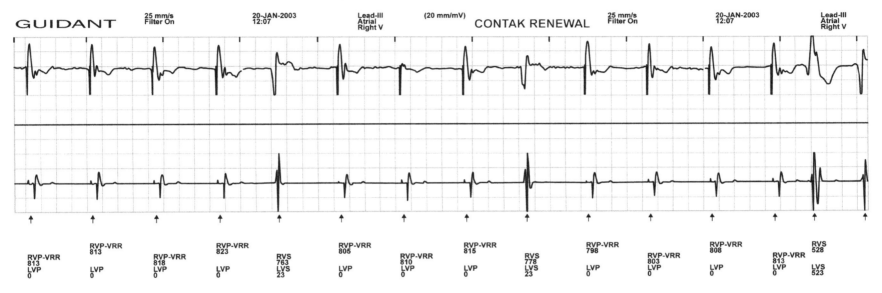

Figure 62.1 Patient's tracing.

Q:

What is the cause of the variation in ventricular pacing intervals from 798 to 823 ms?

1. Inappropriate tracing of AF
2. Ventricular Rate Regulation (VRR)
3. Rate smoothing
4. AV search hysteresis
5. Managed Ventricular Pacing

62

2. Ventricular Rate Regulation (VRR)

A common reason for requesting evaluation of a potentially malfunctioning device is the in-hospital observation of varying pacing rates above the set lower rate. While rate responsive sensor-driven pacing is the most common reason for this, in some cases, specific device algorithms may be operative.

Atrial fibrillation can influence paced rates in several ways. Mode switch may have occurred, and if recorded on telemetry, the change may cause concern. Several AF suppression algorithms (atrial preference pacing, atrial dynamic overdrive pacing) ensure paced atrial rates faster than the base rate to suppress triggers of AF. With post mode switch overdrive pacing (Medtronic), the atrial rates are increased soon after a termination of AF is detected to prevent early recurrence of AF. In addition to such arrhythmia suppression algorithms, more commonly,

algorithms designed to create irregular ventricular rate during AF (Conducted Atrial Fibrillation Response, Medtronic; ventricular rate regularization, Boston Scientific) may be programmed on.

In Figure 62.2, VRR is programmed on (circled) and annotated. VRR and similar algorithms are designed to reduce VV cycle length variation during AF with antegrade conduction. When operative, there is less irregularity, a sometimes troublesome cause of symptoms in patients, particularly those with valvular heart disease.

Rate smoothing (answer 3; Boston Scientific) has a similar goal in preventing marked variation in heart rate but is operative during non-mode-switched episodes as a response to ectopy and sudden intrinsic rate changes. Continued irregularity either from rapidly conducted AF or PVCs will still occur if they do so with close coupling intervals.

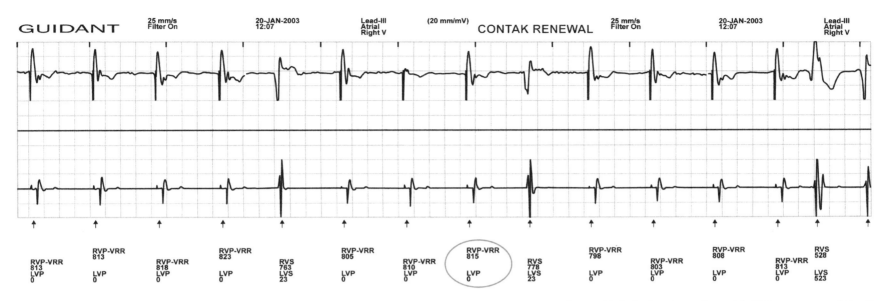

Figure 62.2 Patient's tracing with VRR programmed "on."

62

The ECG in Figure 62.3 is obtained from a patient with AF and a biventricular pacing device (Boston Scientific).

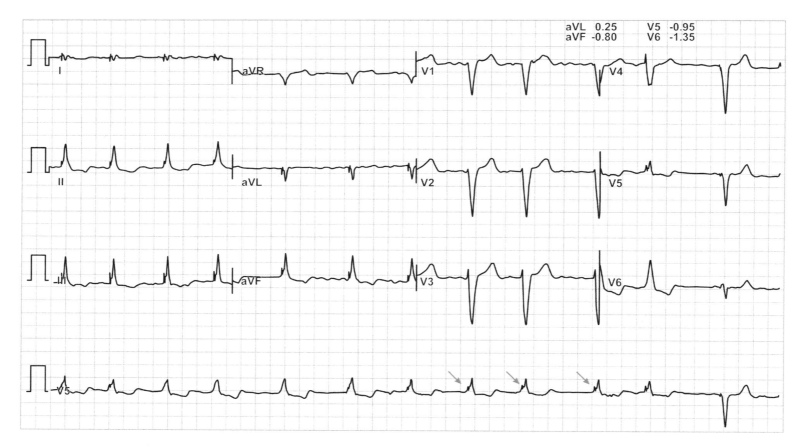

Figure 62.3 Patient's tracing.

Q: *What is the cause of the pacing spikes (arrows) occurring after the onset of the QRS complex?*

1. Ventricular undersensing

2. Failure to mode switch

3. Atrial undersensing

4. Biventricular triggered pacing

62

4. Biventricular triggered pacing

Several algorithms have been developed to promote biventricular pacing in patients with cardiomyopathy and AF and with antegrade conduction. Biventricular trigger (Boston Scientific) aims to promote interventricular synchrony by pacing the right and left ventricles immediately after a sensed RV event. Since this occurs only after a sensed event on the RV lead, the pacing spike will appear after the onset of the QRS complex. If this is observed in a single beat, ventricular undersensing cannot be excluded, but the timing of the spikes relative to the QRS onset noted on several beats suggests that undersensing is not the issue. Note that the patient will still experience an irregular rhythm, albeit with better synchronization when pacing occurs.

The ECG in Figure 62.4 is from the same patient but with VRR now programmed on. Note that stable biventricular pacing with constant rates and degree of resynchronization is present. A tradeoff with such programming, however, is that the average daily heart rate will typically now be higher, which in turn may give rise to symptoms of ischemia or ventricular dysfunction in some cases. Several other algorithms and conditions may be associated with apparent increased pacing rates:

- Ventricular rate stabilization (VRS, Medtronic) increases the rate (shortens the VA interval in dual-chamber devices) in response to a sensed PVC to decrease patient symptoms and possibly the propensity for arrhythmia.
- Rate-Drop Response (Medtronic) is a feature that may have been enabled in patients with neurocardiogenic syndrome where sensed decreased atrial rates will give rise to increased pacing in an attempt to offset symptoms from low cardiac output in such patients.

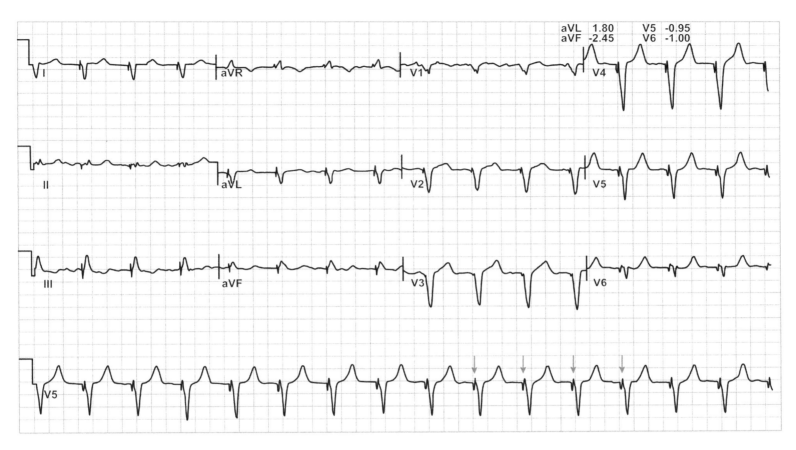

| aVL | 1.80 | V5 | -0.95 |
| aVF | -2.45 | V6 | -1.00 |

Figure 62.4 Patient's ECG, with VVR programmed "on."

62

The tracing in Figure 62.5 was obtained in a patient with a dual-chamber St. Jude Medical device.

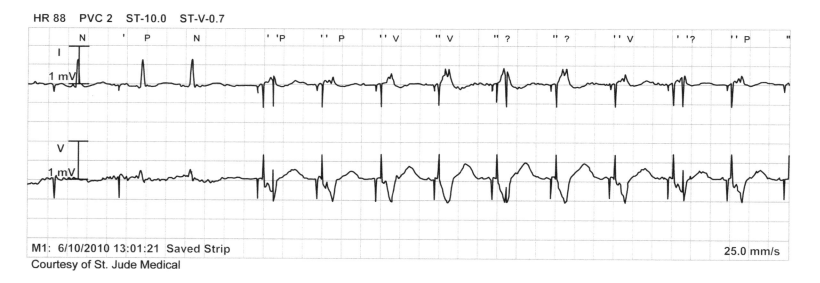

Figure 62.5 Patient's tracing.

Q: *What is the principal finding in this telemetry tracing?*

1. Normal function of mode switch

2. Inappropriate failure to mode switch

3. Normal auto capture test performance

4. Auto capture test with inappropriate detection of loss of capture

62

4. Auto capture test with inappropriate detection of loss of capture

At the beginning of the tracing in Figure 62.6, (1) atrial pacing with antegrade AV nodal conduction is noted. Then (2), the auto capture test is initiated, and atrial pacing with ventricular pacing at a very short (50 ms) AV interval is seen (3). Auto capture and related algorithms allow savings of battery life by generally pacing at a minimum but safe output. The device diagnoses capture by looking at the evoked potential following pacing and capture. If this evoked response is seen, then capture at that output is diagnosed. If, however, the evoked response is not seen, then a backup safety pulse is delivered.

In Figure 62.6, what is the third spike (arrows)? Does this represent normal function? When the device does not sense an evoked response, then a backup pulse is delivered to prevent a ventricular pause. In this tracing, however, clearly, there is ventricular capture, and the backup pulse should not have occurred. This is a result of inappropriate detection of loss of capture. Potential causes for this include difficulty in discerning between a prominent polarization and the evoked response or the occurrence of fusion beats and change in the evoked response vector. In rare cases, an evoked response may be present without ventricular depolarization (exit block despite local capture).

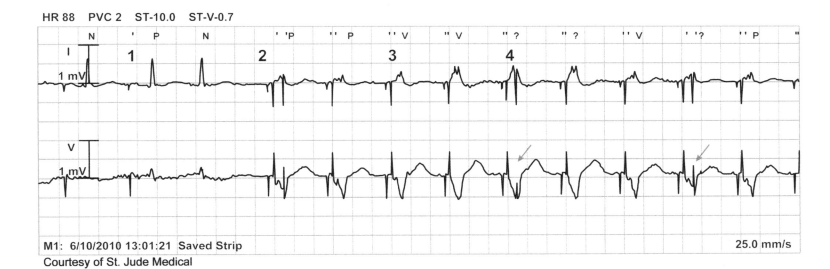

HR 88   PVC 2   ST-10.0   ST-V-0.7

M1: 6/10/2010 13:01:21 Saved Strip

25.0 mm/s

Courtesy of St. Jude Medical

Figure 62.6 Annotated tracing.

62

Additional, unexpected, and closely separated spikes may be seen in other instances as well. Figure 62.7 is obtained from a patient with AF, AV nodal ablation, and a biventricular pacing system.

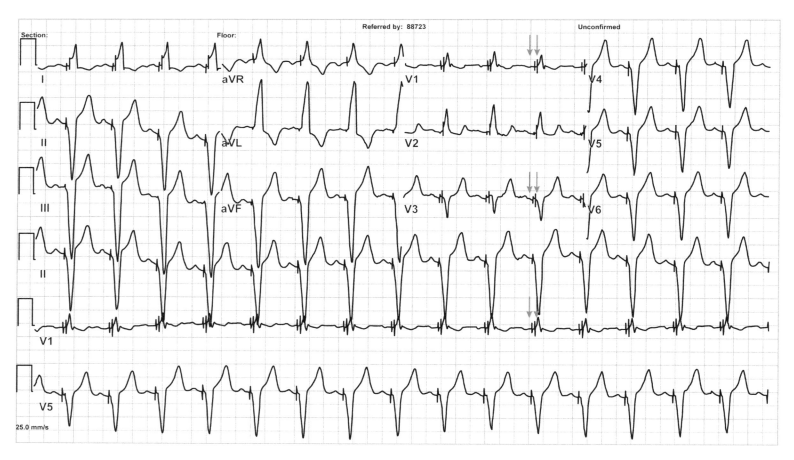

Figure 62.7 Patient's tracing with closely spaced spikes marked.

: *What is the cause of the closely spaced spikes (arrows)?*

1. Failed auto capture test
2. Runaway pacemaker
3. Artifact
4. Programmed left or right ventricular lead offset

62

4. Programmed left or right ventricular lead offset

The patient's chest x-ray is shown in Figure 62.8. The LV lead appears to be in a posterolateral vein about midway between the base and apex, generally a good site for resynchronization. However, in patients with disease of the LV free wall, prominent exit delay from pacing may occur, and when biventricular stimulation is programmed on, the RV lead dominates the wavefront of depolarization, and, in effect, single-chamber pacing results. An offset programmed for the LV lead (LV earlier than RV) will often solve this problem and allow true resynchronization.

When a significant offset is programmed on, 2 distinct spikes for biventricular stimulation (in this case, LV pacing spike first, then RV pacing spike) will be seen.

The Holter monitor tracing shown in Figure 62.9 was obtained in a patient with congenital heart disease and complete heart block. The patient had an endocardial VDD system placed, and ventricular lead auto capture is programmed on.

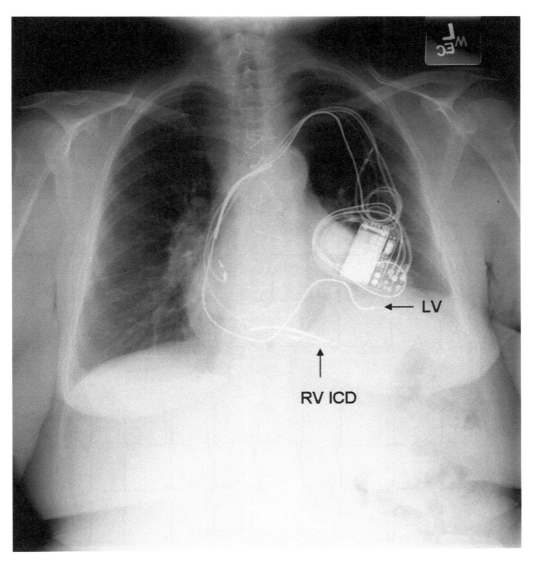

Figure 62.8 Patient's chest x-ray, AP view.

62

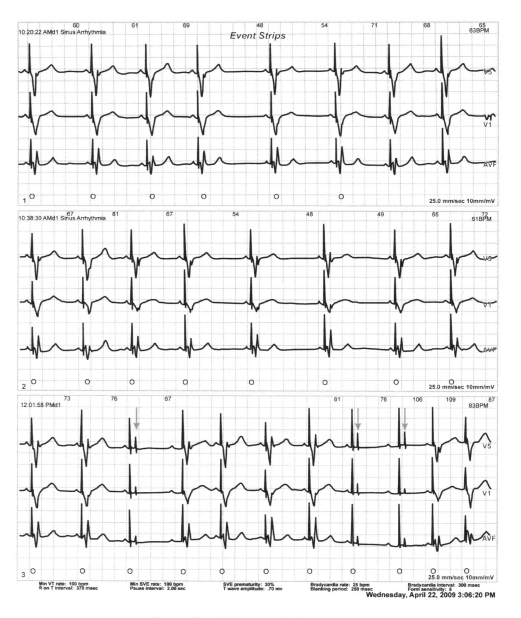

Figure 62.9 Holter monitoring tracing.

Q: *Which of the following is correct?*

1. Ventricular safety pacing
2. VDD pacing with failure to sense in the atrium
3. Normal auto capture function
4. Elevated pacing thresholds with "failure to capture"

62

4. Elevated pacing thresholds with "failure to capture"

What do the 2 spikes (Figure 62.9, arrows) represent? With auto capture programmed on the ventricular lead (patient does not have a pacing system or atrial pacing is possible) includes the first pacing stimulus at a short AV interval and then a search for a ventricular evoked response. If the ventricular evoked response is not found (assumed failure to capture), then the backup pace (second spike) is delivered. Failing to capture from the first spike would be expected as the threshold is being checked. However, the backup spike should capture (programmable output) and failure to do so suggests elevated pacing thresholds.

Figure 62.10 shows the intracardiac EGMs and markers during a ventricular capture test. Note the difference on the V bipolar (circled) when there is failure to capture. The polarization artifact (black arrow) continues to be seen without the evoked response (red arrow).

Apparent failure to capture can be difficult to troubleshoot without an appreciation of any capture management/auto capture algorithms that have been programmed on.

Several types include atrial capture management, RV lead capture management (RV lead capture assurance, Medtronic), and LV lead capture management (Medtronic).

As explained previously, ventricular capture management/assurance involves analysis of the evoked EGM immediately after a stimulus. With appropriate blanking for polarization and decay, capture is assumed when the evoked response is seen.

Atrial capture verification is a relatively simple algorithm where when intrinsic AV nodal conduction is present, the atrium is paced with a long AV interval to look for sensed ventricular events, and the threshold is subsequently checked.

LV capture management is a far more complex algorithm since intrinsic conduction and LV-RV conduction time must be taken into consideration. When the patient is monitored during an LV capture management algorithm, an understanding of the observation should be based on the steps involved:

1. Confirmation of rate stability
2. LV pacing for 4 cycles with an AV delay of 30 ms (no real chance for antegrade AV conduction)
3. Estimation of the interval between the LV stimulus and sensed V on the RV lead (LV-RV conduction time)
4. Pacing with an AV delay equal to the LV-RV conduction time plus 80 ms to confirm that intrinsic conduction will not interfere with LV threshold testing
5. Finally, delivery of LV test pulses and LV capture confirmation if the RV sensed event falls within the window surrounding the predetermined LV-RV conduction time.

Capture management is typically done at 1 am, and interestingly, some patients may wake up at that time and note the test being performed possibly from phrenic nerve stimulation at the higher outputs.

In summary, a thorough knowledge of common device algorithms that may present with apparent inappropriate rapid pacing, variance in AV intervals, and loss of capture need to be understood to adequately evaluate patients with device "malfunction."

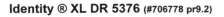

Identity ® XL DR 5376 (#706778 pr9.2)

Ventricular Capture Test

Today: **3.38 v** @ 1.0 ms(Uni)

Last session: 3.25 V @ 1.0 ms(Uni)

Apr 17, 2009 2:01 pm (Sweep Speed: 25 mm/s)

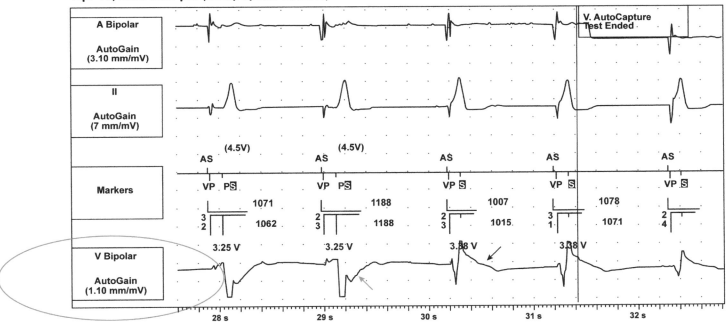

Figure 62.10 Intracardiac EGMs and markers.

Case 63

In patients with a CRT device, the 12-lead ECG yields important information on analysis.

63

Which of the following best states the underlying principle that allows ECG-based localization of pacing site and resynchronization?

1. When the vector of activation moves toward the positive pole of the ECG lead, an R wave is generated
2. When the vector of activation moves toward the positive pole of the ECG lead, an S wave is generated
3. The chest leads cannot be used for pacing site localization
4. Only the pectoral leads can be used for ECG localization
5. None of the above

63

1. When the vector of activation moves toward the positive pole of the ECG lead, an R wave is generated

The premise for electrocardiographic analysis and troubleshooting resynchronization devices is based on this principle. Thus, knowing the positive pole for any ECG lead and observing whether predominantly an R wave or S wave is generated will quickly allow fairly detailed localization of the likely pacing site. For example, the positive pole for lead I is in the left arm. Thus, RV pacing where the vector will move from the right toward the left will result in an R wave in lead I.

The chest leads can be used along with the limb leads for analysis. The location of these leads (V_1-V_6) serves as the "positive" pole, and thus, lead V_1 is negative with most RV pacing (vector moving away from V_1) and positive with most LV pacing sites (vector moving from LV toward the RV).

The ECG in Figure 63.1 was obtained from a patient with dilated cardiomyopathy following cardiac resynchronization device implantation.

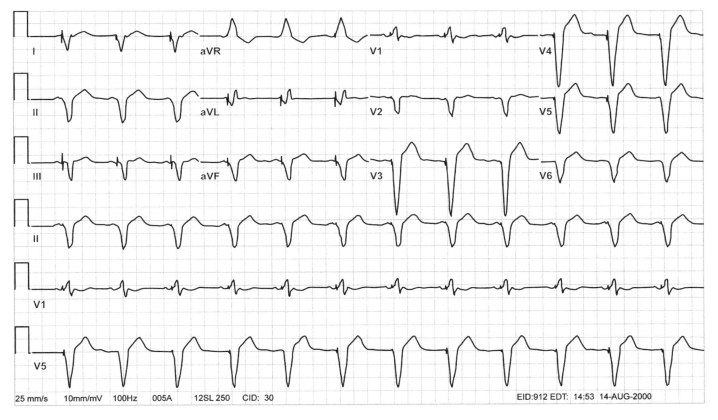

63

Figure 63.1 Patient's ECG.

Which of the following observations is correct?

Q:

1. ECG is consistent with RV only pacing
2. The ECG suggests LV pacing from the anterior interventricular vein
3. There is failure to capture from the LV lead
4. The ECG is consistent with biventricular pacing with an LV lead placed in the posterolateral venous system
5. None of the above

63

4. The ECG is consistent with biventricular pacing with an LV lead placed in the posterolateral venous system

When analyzing this ECG, we should first determine whether this is likely RV or LV pacing. There is a clear prominent R wave in lead V_1 (RBBB morphology), and, in addition, lead I has a prominent S wave (left to right activation). Thus, the pacing site clearly involves stimulation of the left ventricle. We can further surmise that biventricular stimulation is occurring given the relatively narrow QRS. The LV site likely involves the posterior lateral segments since there are QS complexes in II-aVF (posterior/inferior stimulation) and all negative in lead I (lateral stimulation).

The corresponding left anterior oblique radiograph of the LV lead position in this patient is shown in Figure 63.2. This is a typical position for CRT device LV lead implant, and this, along with other sites on the LV free wall about midway from the base to apex are considered optimal sites for LV lead placement.

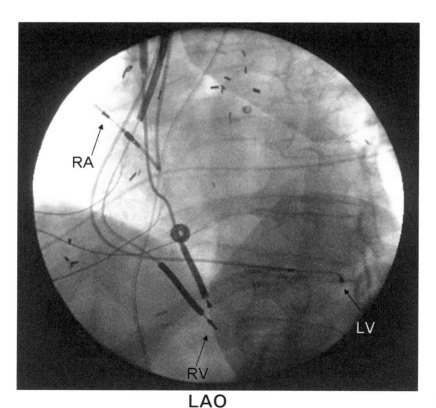

Figure 63.2 Radiograph of LV lead position.

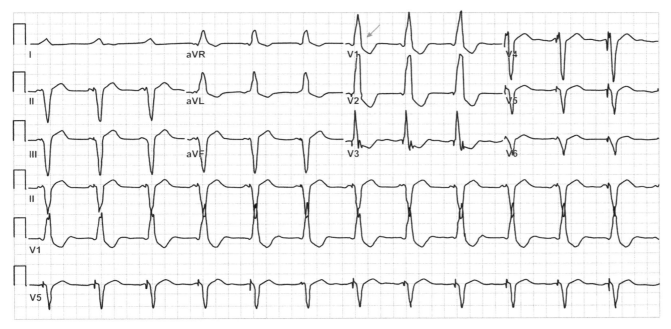

63

Figure 63.3 Patient's ECG.

The ECG obtained in Figure 63.3 during LV lead stimulation is most consistent with the LV lead being in which vein-related position?

Q:

1. Middle cardiac vein
2. Anterior interventricular vein
3. Posterolateral vein
4. Any of the above
5. None of the above

63

1. Middle cardiac vein

The very prominent R wave in V$_1$ (Figure 63.3, arrow) strongly suggests LV stimulation. Leads II, III, and aVF are all negative (S waves) consistent with inferior/posterior LV stimulation (superior axis) and thus excluding anterior interventricular vein pacing. There is an R wave in lead I; thus, there is a significant vector of activation toward the left, consistent with septal LV stimulation. These features are most consistent with middle cardiac vein pacing.

Figure 63.4 is obtained with RV stimulation. Note that if one did not look at the precordial leads, there is very little to distinguish between middle cardiac vein (Figure 63.5) and RV (Figure 63.4) stimulation. The reason for this is that the middle cardiac vein runs in the posterior interventricular groove and is essentially the leftward neighbor of the posterior right ventricle. The middle cardiac vein itself is generally not an ideal site for pacing the left ventricle, but several lateral venous branches often exist, and the posterolateral or lateral LV wall can be reached via this vein.

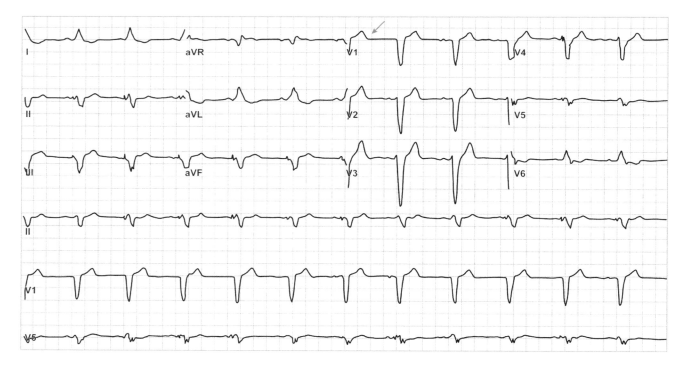

Figure 63.4 Tracing obtained with RV stimulation.

63

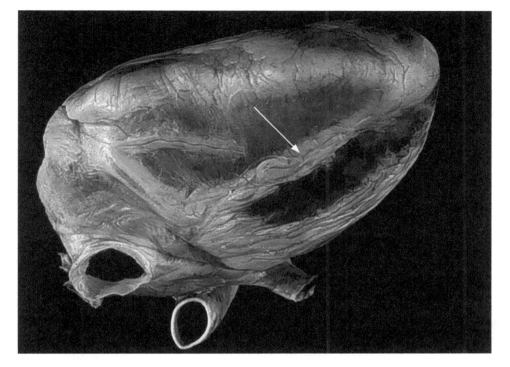

Figure 63.5 Middle cardiac vein (MCV).

In which of the following situations might middle cardiac vein cannulation and use for LV stimulation be considered?

1. Coronary sinus dissection
2. Prominent Vieussens valve
3. Patient with corrected transposition of the great vessels
4. All of the above
5. None of the above

63

4. All of the above

The middle cardiac vein can be used to access the LV free wall whenever the mid or distal coronary sinus is difficult to access.

Figure 63.6 shows the right and left anterior oblique (RAO, LAO) views of a coronary sinus angiogram. The arrow points to a prominent Vieussens valve that "guards" the opening of the posterolateral/lateral vein. In situations like this or with mid coronary sinus stenosis, dissec-tion, etc, the proximally located middle cardiac vein can be cannulated and the lead threaded through one of its lateral branches.

There are, however, important exceptions to the general rule that RBBB morphology with pacing equals LV and LBBB morphology equals RV.

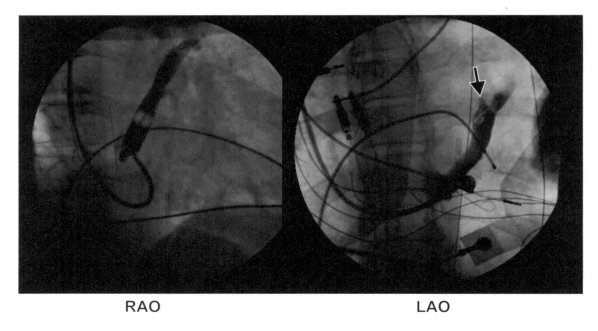

RAO   LAO

Figure 63.6 Right and left anterior oblique (RAO, LAO) views of coronary sinus angiogram.

The 12-lead ECG shown in Figure 63.7 was obtained from a patient with chronic obstructive pulmonary disease and dilated cardiomyopathy with RV pacing only. There is a significant R wave in lead V_1. With very apical locations in patients with counterclockwise rotated hearts, the pacing site is sufficiently apical to and leftward of lead V_1 location that an R wave can be generated yet the lead is located in the RV. Note, however, that lead I is positive, signifying a significant right-to-left activation wavefront consistent with RV pacing.

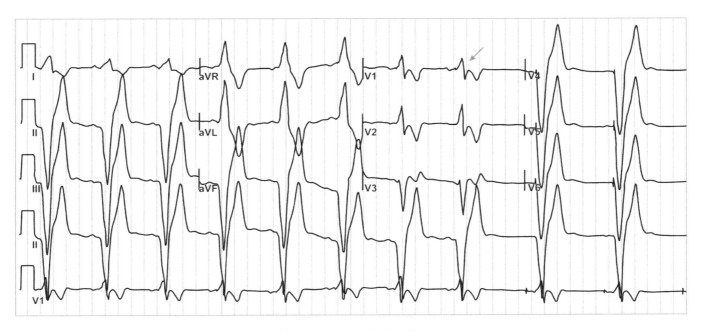

Figure 63.7 Patient's ECG.

63

Figure 63.8 was obtained from a patient with LV lead stimulation only. There is clearly an LBBB morphology pattern; however, this lead was located in the vicinity of the anterior interventricular vein near the interventricular septum. Thus, there is a strong inferior axis (R waves in leads II, III, and aVF) and a negative deflection in lead I (arrow shows start of LV pacing). RV outflow tract pacing may also produce a very similar and essentially indistinguishable QRS morphology (RV outflow tract pacing in the vicinity of the pulmonic valve).

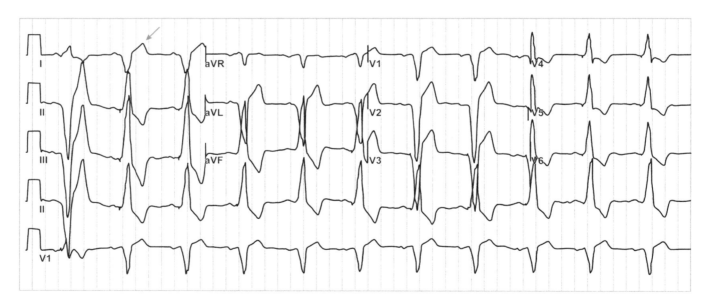

Figure 63.8 Patient's ECG with LV lead stimulation only.

63

Although analyzing the ECG can readily help identify the specific site of pacing, a very important utility of detailed ECG analysis lies in assessing the degree of synchronous biventricular electrical activation.

The 12-lead ECG shown in Figure 63.9 is obtained from a patient with advanced cardiomyopathy and during RV lead only stimulation, the LBBB pattern and R wave in lead I are consistent with this pacing site location.

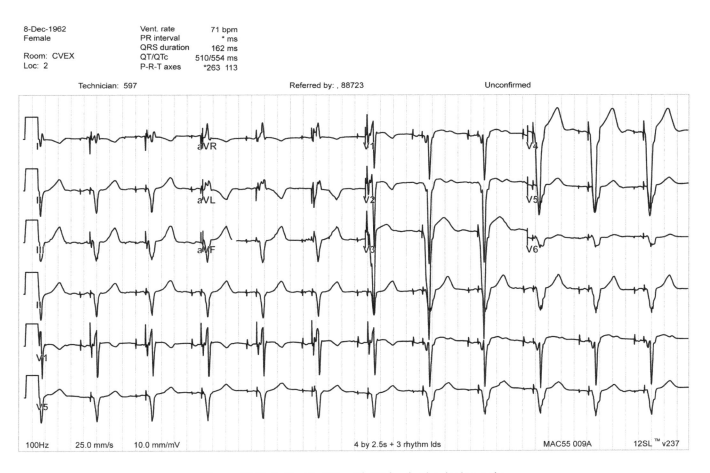

Figure 63.9 Patient's ECG with RV lead stimulation only.

63

In the same patient, Figure 63.10 shows pacing from the LV lead that was located on the lateral LV free wall. There is a very tall R wave in lead V_1 characteristic of LV pacing and a QS pattern in lead I.

Figure 63.11 is the ECG from the same patient with simultaneous biventricular stimulation. One can readily note that the QRS morphol-

ogy with *biventricular* stimulation is almost identical to what was seen with RV site stimulation alone.

One may even consider that the LV lead is nonfunctional; however, as seen in Figure 63.10, LV lead pacing was normal and with good thresholds. Why is LV lead site stimulation not seen with simultaneous biven-

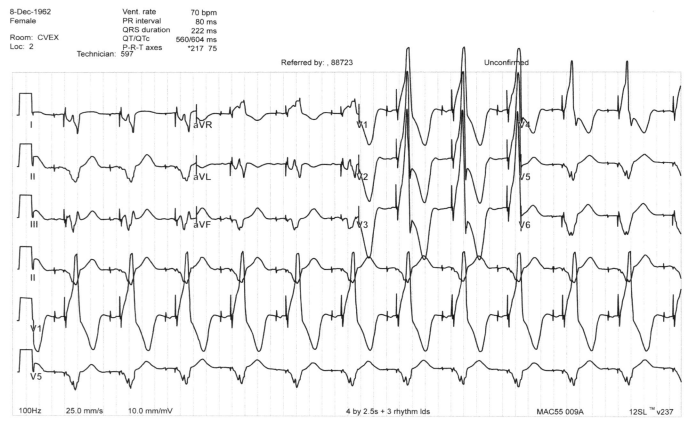

Figure 63.10 ECG showing pacing from LV lead located on lateral LV free wall.

tricular pacing? In patients with very diseased LV myocardium, there can be significant exit delay via zones of viable but slowly conducting tissue from the LV free wall site. In this situation, with simultaneous pacing, the bulk of the myocardium is activated from the RV lead before there is a chance for LV stimulation to exit from the diseased myocardium.

In Figure 63.12, an offset has been programmed for the LV lead to try to negate the effect of this exit delay. We note a slightly more LV-like vector is now found with lead I being completely negative. With this programmed LV offset, evidence of biventricular stimulation and electrical synchrony (features of RV and LV lead pacing) are seen.

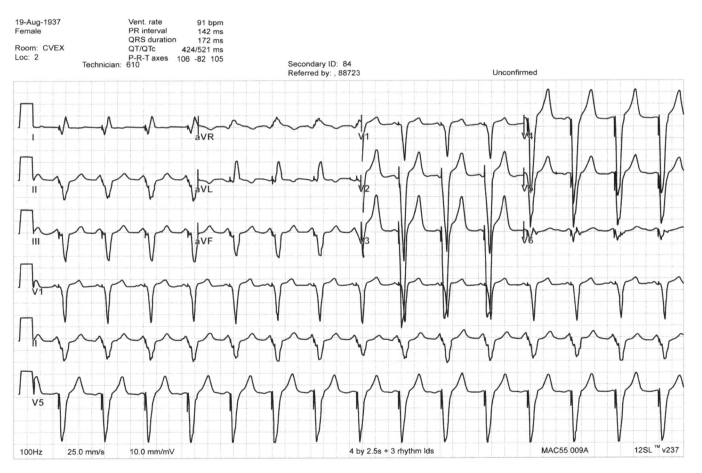

Figure 63.11 Patient's ECG with simultaneous biventricular stimulation.

63

Figure 63.13 is obtained from a patient with prior myocardial infarction and symptomatic congestive heart failure with a biventricular ICD in place. The LV lead is placed in an anterolateral vein, and the RV lead is in the region of the RV apex.

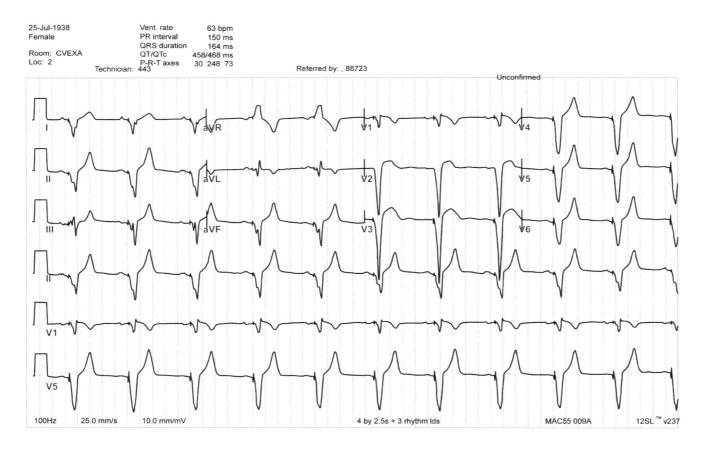

Figure 63.12 ECG showing an offset programmed for LV lead.

63

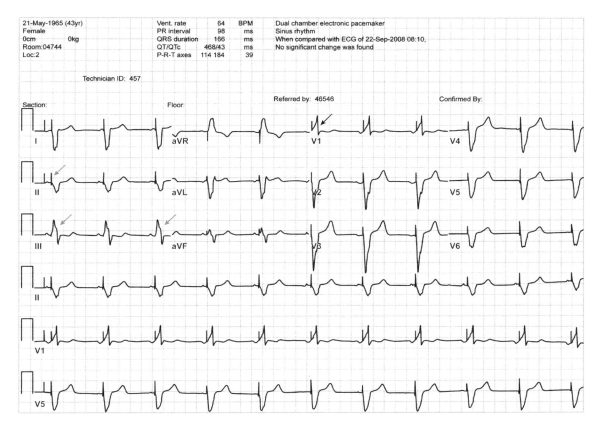

Figure 63.13 ECG with biventricular ICD in place.

21-May-1965 (43yr)   Vent. rate   64   BPM   Dual chamber electronic pacemaker
Female   PR interval   98   ms   Sinus rhythm
0cm   0kg   QRS duration 166   ms   When compared with ECG of 22-Sep-2008 08:10,
Room:04744   QT/QTc   468/43   ms   No significant change was found
Loc:2   P-R-T axes 114 184 39

Technician ID: 457

Section: Floor: Referred by: 46546   Confirmed By:

Q: Which of the following is likely true with regard to biventricular synchronous pacing?

1. The pacing vector is most consistent with LV lead pacing only

2. The LV lead is nonfunctional

3. A strong LV offset should be considered (LV earlier than RV)

4. There is evidence of biventricular pacing

63

4. There is evidence of biventricular pacing

There is a definite R wave in lead V_1 (black arrow) consistent with LV stimulation. However, the inferior leads (red arrows) show a mixed pattern with a QS complex in lead II and a significant R wave in lead III. Since we are given the knowledge that the LV lead is in the anterolateral position, we would expect a relatively strong inferior axis (R wave in lead II). Thus, there is a significant contribution from the RV apical lead as well. In total, the ECG is consistent with biventricular stimulation with a suitably programmed offset.

It should be emphasized, however, that ECG analysis for resynchronization is only reflective of the adequacy of biventricular *electrical* stimulation. In patients with diseased hearts and abnormal and variable electromechanical coupling intervals and/or multiple myocardial infarc-tions, there can be marked mechanical dyssynchronous ventricular activation despite reasonable electrical synchrony. While this limitation must be kept in mind for ECG analysis, if on the ECG there is no evidence of LV stimulation despite biventricular pacing one cannot expect any benefit from the LV lead implantation.

Figure 63.14 is a 12-lead ECG obtained from a patient with a biventricular system and the LV pacing vector between the LV tip (cathode) and RV ring (anode). The LV lead is in the posterolateral wall, and the RV lead is in the RV apex. Figure 63.14 is obtained with LV pacing output just above threshold, and Figure 63.15 (with identical stimulation sites and offset) at high output pacing.

63

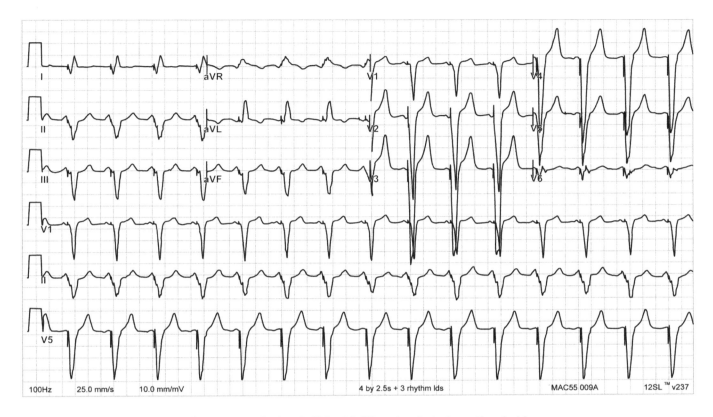

100Hz   25.0 mm/s   10.0 mm/mV   4 by 2.5s + 3 rhythm lds   MAC55 009A   12SL ™ v237

Figure 63.14 Patient's ECG with LV pacing just above threshold.

63

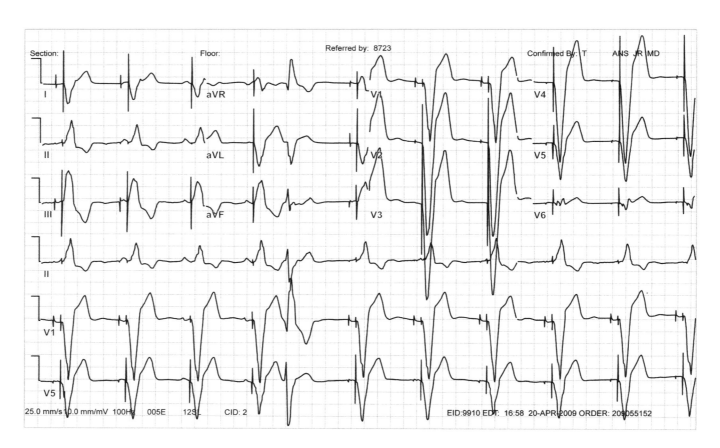

Figure 63.15 Patient's ECG with high output pacing.

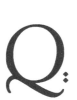

Which of the following may be a reason in this patient (Figures 63.14 and 63.15) for failure of response to resynchronization therapy?

1. Suboptimal LV lead placement

2. Anodal stimulation

3. Frequent PVCs

4. Possible AV dyssynchrony

5. All of the above

63

5. All of the above

A complete analysis of the ECGs may provide important clues as to why a patient may not be achieving maximal benefit from a CRT device. With Figure 63.15, we note a marked change in the pacing vector although the lead location and offset were unchanged. The phenomenon where pacing vector varies with output and typically with LV configuration with cathode being the LV tip and anode the RV coil or ring is called anodal stimulation. The stimulation wavefront is from the RV ring when anodal stimulation occurs, generally negating the potential benefits of LV site stimulation.

We also note frequent PVCs have developed (possibly related to the slower pacing rate in Figure 63.15). This may also be a cause of functional deterioration by various mechanisms including worsening of cardiomyopathy, inhibition of pacing, and AV dyssynchrony.

With the programmed AV interval, we note that ventricular stimulation appears to occur even before the termination of the P wave (Figure 63.15). The ECG analysis for AV synchrony, however, is limited since the key mechanical interval involves left atrial–left ventricular mechanical synchrony. Even when surface ECG-based AV intervals appear opti-

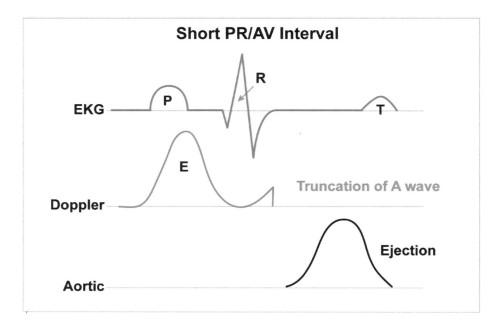

Figure 63.16 Short PR/AV interval.

mal when there is significant interatrial conduction delay, inappropriate mechanical left AV-LV timings may result.

As noted in Figure 63.16, when there is a short AV (PR) interval, LV contraction occurs before completion of left atrial emptying, "truncating" the atrial filling wave noted with mitral valve pulse wave Doppler imaging.

On the other hand, as seen in Figure 63.17, with a very prolonged programmed AV interval, left atrial emptying has completed, but since LV contraction still doesn't start, early closure of the mitral valve and possible diastolic mitral regurgitation may occur and some patients associated with signs of worsening LV failure.

Thus, although adjunctive ECG and overall clinical evaluation (worsening coronary disease, etc.) must all be considered when troubleshooting resynchronization failure, important clues from the ECG when appropriately analyzed are an additional tool available for the device and heart failure physician.

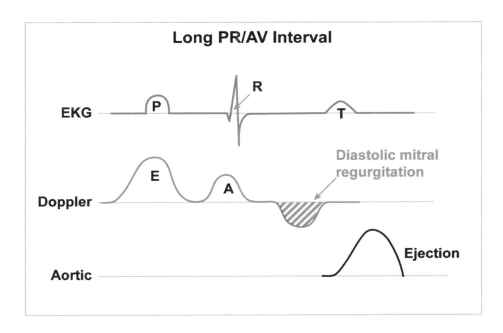

Figure 63.17 Long PR/AV interval.

Case 64

A patient with a dual-chamber ICD presents with palpitations. Figure 64.1 shows the remote monitoring data obtained coincident with a long episode of palpitations.

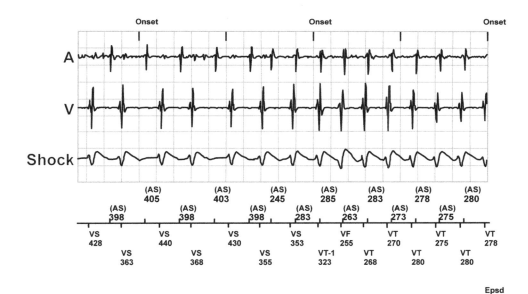

Figure 64.1 Patient's monitoring data.

Q: *What is the likely mechanism of tachycardia?*

1. Ventricular tachycardia
2. AV node reentrant tachycardia
3. Atrial fibrillation
4. Sinus tachycardia

64

2. AV node reentrant tachycardia

As seen in Figure 64.2, the initiating beat of tachycardia is likely a premature atrial complex (PAC, arrow). Following this beat, there is a relatively long AV interval and then initiation of the tachyarrhythmia. The shock EGM (far-field) morphology is relatively similar to that seen in sinus rhythm.

Following the PAC initiation, the tachycardia has near-simultaneous activation of the atrial and ventricular EGMs. These features strongly suggest AVNRT as the likely mechanism of tachycardia.

Less frequently, atrial tachycardia may present with simultaneous atrial and ventricular EGMs with one atrial beat conducting with significant AV delay to produce the next ventricular EGM, which coincidently occurs at the same time as the next atrial tachycardia beat. This situation is rarely sustained but along with AVNRT, junctional tachycardia, and ventricular tachycardia with long stable retrograde VA activation can present as tachycardia with simultaneous ventricle and atrial EGMs. By far the most likely clinical arrhythmia among this group is AVNRT.

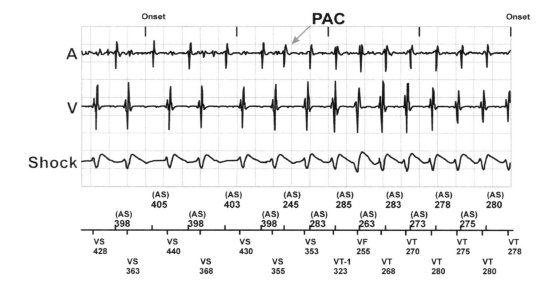

Figure 64.2 Premature atrial contraction (PAC).

64

Figure 64.3 shows a series of similar tracings. Is ICD therapy appropriate in these instances?

Once again we note in Figure 64.3 that the tachycardia initiates with rapid atrial activity and periods where there are more atrial EGMs than ventricular EGMs, suggesting a supraventricular tachycardia, possibly early AF. Note, the far-field ventricular EGMs change in morphology. This is not uncommon with bundle branch aberrancy seen during AF.

At the beginning of the tracing shown in Figure 64.4, the patient is likely in sinus rhythm. Note the small far-field ventricular EGM on the atrial channel. There are premature ventricular beats, the first occurring

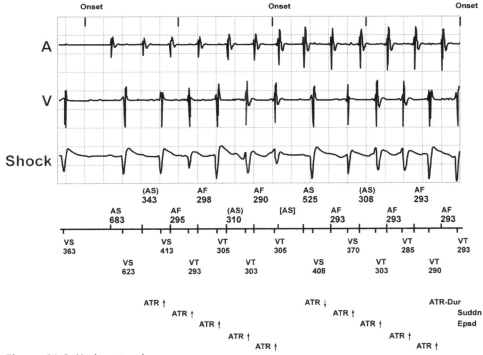

Figure 64.3 Various tracings.

64

soon after the atrial EGM and too soon to represent AV conduction and then the second beat (arrow) clearly ventricular in origin with no preceding atrial EGM. Although once tachycardia stabilizes, it can be difficult to distinguish antegrade versus retrograde 1:1 conduction. The initiation would clearly establish the diagnosis as ventricular tachycardia and ICD treatment as appropriate.

In the tracing shown in Figure 64.5, prior to initiation of the ventricular tachyarrhythmia, the patient is in a stable atrial tachyarrhythmia with slow AV conduction. If one were only to look at the right-hand side of this tracing, it would not be easy to define the mechanism of tachycardia and the simultaneous presence of atrial and ventricular tachycardias. The gradual "frame-shifting" as a result of the slight difference (15 ms) in the cycle lengths of the 2 tachycardias would have been a clue. However, looking at the initiation of tachycardia with preexisting atrial tachycardia, slow AV nodal conduction (thus excluding rapid antegrade conduction), and the distinct change in the ventricular EGM morphology, all would clearly allow diagnosis of dual tachycardia and appropriate therapy for the recent onset ventricular tachycardia.

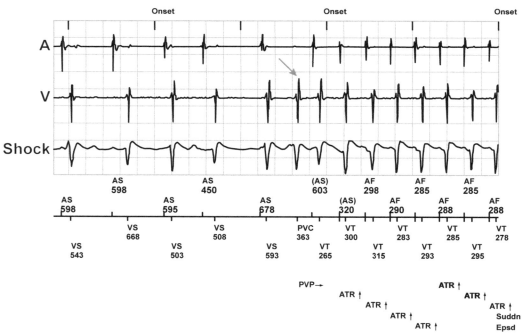

Figure 64.4 Annotated tracings.

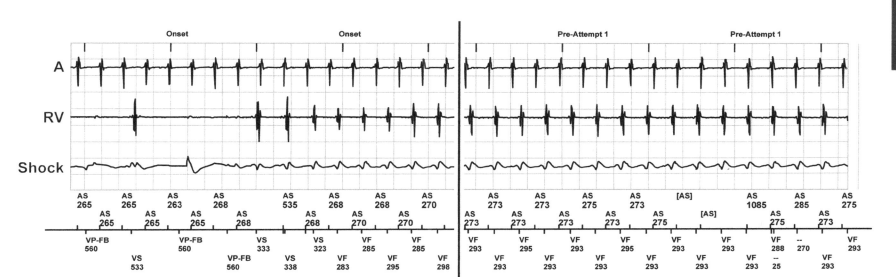

Figure 64.5 Tracing prior to initiation of the ventricular tachyarrhythmia.

64

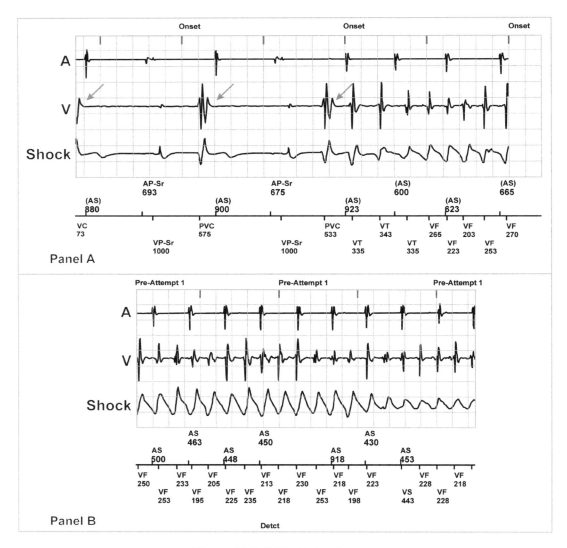

Figure 64.6 Patient's tracings.

Q: *In the tracings shown in Figure 64.6, which of the following observations are accurate?*

1. A monomorphic ventricular tachycardia is present
2. Ventricular fibrillation is present
3. A supraventricular tachycardia is present
4. Frequent PVCs with triggering of polymorphic ventricular tachycardia is noted

64

4. Frequent PVCs with triggering of polymorphic ventricular tachycardia is noted

At the beginning of Figure 64.6 (panel A), the patient is in an AP-VP paced rhythm with PVCs. Following one of the PVCs, a polymorphic ventricular tachycardia is initiated. The PVCs themselves are likely monomorphic with very similar near-field and far-field EGMs and also similar timing between the near-field and far-field EGMs. This type of initiation is important to recognize since radiofrequency ablation could be considered targeting the PVCs to prevent recurrent frequent shocks.

Observation of the arrhythmia itself (panel B) without knowledge of the initiating sequence would not allow such determinations.

In Figure 64.7, once again PVCs are noted. Retrograde conduction likely occurs through one of the PVCs, producing a transient atrial arrhythmia. The PVCs also induce a stable monomorphic ventricular tachycardia. The type of initiation seen here would suggest that ablation targeting the PVCs themselves would be of little value, unlike the patient in Figure 64.7. In this instance, if frequent shocks despite medi-

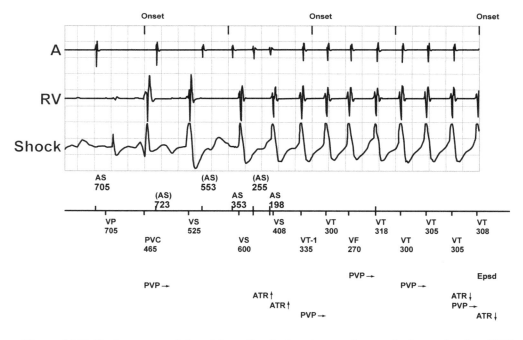

Figure 64.7 Electrograms retrieved from the device show early ventricular activation (PVC) with retrograde conduction to the atrium followed by initiation of ventricular tachycardia.

64

cal therapy continue to occur, a substrate-based ablation targeting the ventricular tachycardia circuit would be the preferred approach.

Figure 64.8 is a continuation of the same arrhythmia seen in Figure 64.7. Note there is now stable VA conduction with near-simultaneous atrial and ventricular EGMs. This often signifies AVNRT, but occasionally, as in this case, when observing a relatively small segment of the arrhythmia, there may be stable VA conduction with coincidental

VT cycle length and VA conduction time giving the appearance of simultaneous VA activation. Observation of the initiating sequence and comparison of the morphology of the shock EGMs with conducted rhythm, if present, will help clarify the issue.

Figure 64.9 was obtained in a patient with tachypalpitation and subsequent ICD therapy and presyncope. The initiation of the arrhythmia is consistent with an SVT process, likely AVNRT. Note, initially

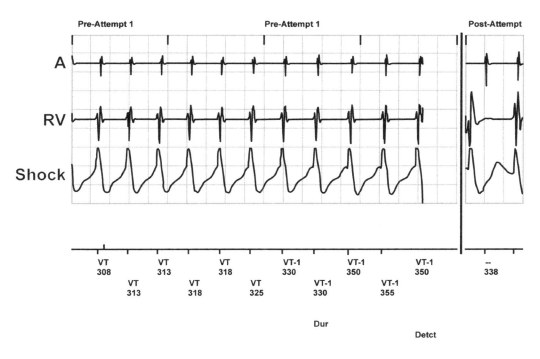

Figure 64.8 Intradevice electrograms during ventricular tachycardia. Earliest activation is on the shock electrograms (far field) with conduction to the atrium in a retrograde 1:1 fashion.

64

there is sinus rhythm with stable atrial ventricular conduction. Premature atrial complexes are seen with a long AV interval following the second PAC (arrow) and then tachycardia with simultaneous VA EGMs. The far-field EGMs are similar to conducted rhythm.

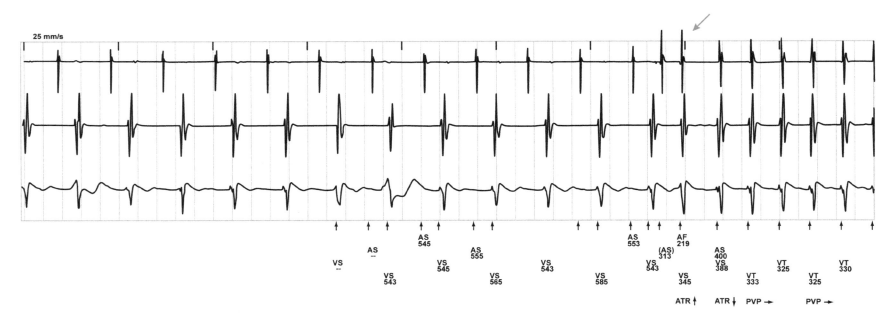

Figure 64.9 Tracing of patient with tachypalpitation.

The tachycardia stabilizes, and the AVNRT is detected in the ventricular tachycardia zone (Figure 64.10).

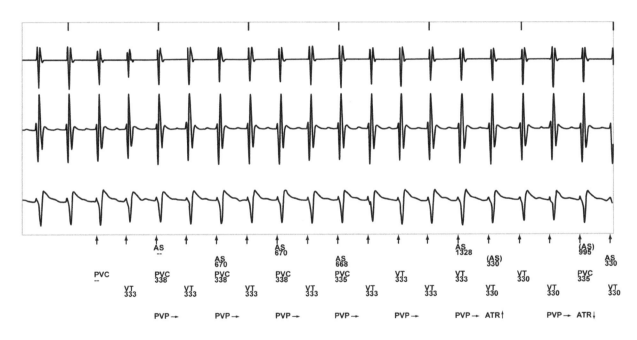

Figure 64.10 Intracardiac EGMs during sustained tachycardia.

64

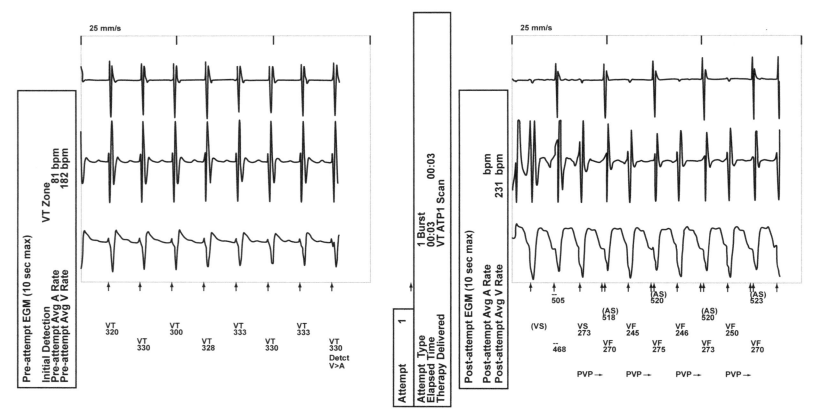

Figure 64.11 Patient's tracings.

Q: *The tachycardia detected at VT triggers antitachycardia pacing. Following ATP, what is the observation seen in Figure 64.11?*

1. AVNRT terminates
2. Ventricular tachycardia is initiated
3. There is a change in the far-field ventricular EGMs
4. All of the above

64

4. All of the above

The antitachycardia pacing, although delivered in the ventricle, may terminate a variety of supraventricular tachycardias including AVNRT. In this instance the ATP simultaneously initiates a ventricular tachycardia with clear preponderance of ventricular EGMs (V > A) and a distinct change in the far-field EGM morphology.

In Figure 64.12, we note persistence of the ventricular tachycardia with VA dissociation.

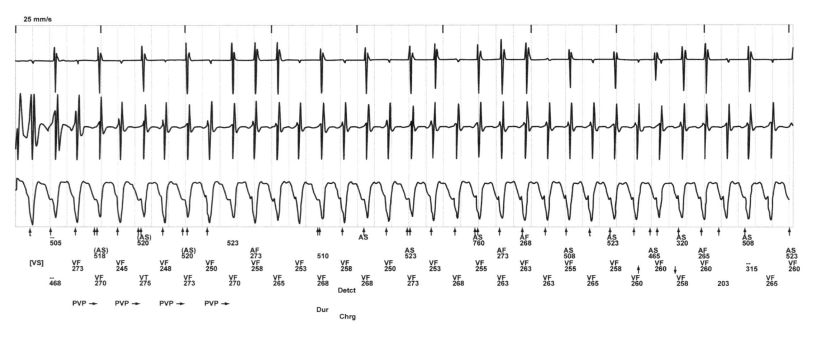

Figure 64.12 Tracing showing ventricular tachycardia with VA dissociation.

64

A subsequent episode of ATP therapy (Figure 64.13) terminates the ventricular tachycardia, and sinus rhythm ensues.

VA simultaneous tachycardias, dual tachycardias, and transition from one tachycardia to another may all present challenges for inter-preting appropriateness of therapy and planning invasive and pharma-cological approaches to prevent shocks. Close scrutiny of initiating and terminating sequences often aids in answering these questions.

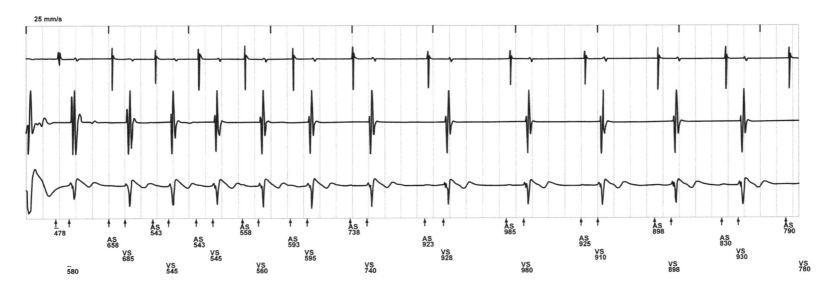

Figure 64.13 Tracing after ATP therapy.

Case 65

Figures 65.1 and 65.2 are tracings obtained from a patient with a Boston Scientific dual-chamber ICD placed for intermittent AV block and ischemic cardiomyopathy. The device is programmed with a sensed AV delay of 150 ms and paced AV delay of 180 ms.

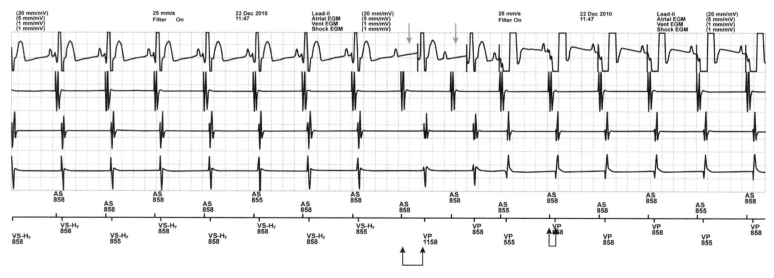

Figure 65.1 Tracing showing varying AV interval.

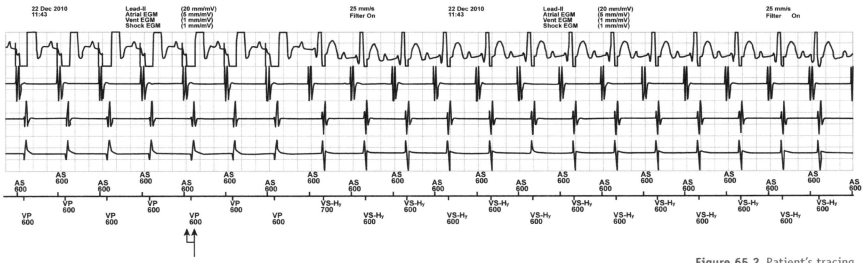

Figure 65.2 Patient's tracing.

Q: *What is the cause of the varying AV interval noticed in Figure 65.1 (black arrows)?*

1. Differential AV interval
2. Rate-adaptive or dynamic AV interval
3. Positive AV search hysteresis
4. Automatic PVARP

65

3. Positive AV search hysteresis

The actual sensed or paced AV intervals may be different from programmed parameters for a number of reasons. Positive AV search hysteresis aims at promoting intrinsic AV conduction in dual-chamber devices and is a common cause of varying AV interval. The specific tracings shown illustrate the AV search + algorithm (Boston Scientific).

At the beginning of the tracing, sensed atrial events are followed by paced ventricular events after the programmed sensed AV event. With this specific AV search hysteresis algorithm, the device progressively extends the AV interval for 8 cycles to determine if sensed ventricular events (VS) will occur. Since a VS occurs, the extended AV interval persists until the AV conduction time exceeds the preset hysteresis AV delay (400 ms in this case) for 2/10 cycles (red arrows). Following this, the device reverts back to the programmed AV intervals (Figure 65.3).

It should be noted with this AV search hysteresis algorithm that AV pacing never occurs *shorter* than the programmed AV interval. Table 65.1 summarizes certain search hysteresis algorithms from specific manufacturers.

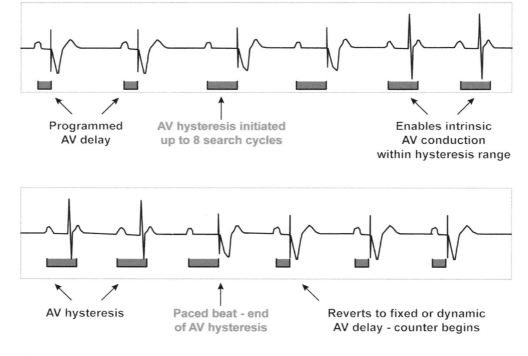

Figure 65.3 AV search hysteresis algorithm.

65

Table 65.1 Manufacturer-Specific AV Hysteresis Programs

MEDTRONIC

Search AV +

The pacemaker analyzes the 16 most recent AV conduction sequences and adjusts the positive AV/sensed AV to keep intrinsic conducted events in an "AV delay window" that precedes scheduled paced events by 15 to 55 ms. The AV delay window is set to promote intrinsic conduction to the ventricles, but ends early enough to avoid fusion or pseudofusion beats if pacing is necessary. The AV conduction times of the 16 most recent AV conduction sequences are measured. If the majority of the sensed events occur within 15 ms of the scheduled ventricular pace or if the majority are paced events, the AV interval is increased by 62 ms for the next 16 cycles. If the sensed events occur more than 55 ms before the scheduled V pace, the AV interval is shortened by 8 ms for the next 16 cycles. Search AV+ is turned off if Managed Ventricular Pacing is programmed on.

BOSTON SCIENTIFIC

AV Search Hysteresis

The AV delay is lengthened periodically after a programmed number of consecutive paced cycles ("AV search interval" 32–1024 cycles) by a programmable percentage ("AV increase" 10%–100%) for up to 8 consecutive cardiac cycles. The hysteresis AV delay will remain active as long as the intrinsic PR intervals are shorter than the hysteresis AV delay. The pacemaker will revert to the programmed AV delay following the first ventricular pace at the hysteresis AV delay, or when the 8-cycle search expires without sensing intrinsic ventricular activity.

AV Search +

Similar to AV search hysteresis, except the pacemaker will revert to programmed AV delay after 2 paced ventricular events occur in 10 cycles, instead of after the first paced event.

ST JUDE MEDICAL

Ventricular Intrinsic Preference Parameter (VIPR)

The VIPR extends the programmed AV delay by a programmed interval ("VIP extension parameter") for a programmed number of cycles ("search cycle's parameter") to search for intrinsic conduction. If an intrinsic event occurs, the extended AV delay remains in effect. If a sensed event does not occur, the programmed AV delay is restored. The "search interval parameter" determines how frequently the device extends the AV interval to search for intrinsic conduction.

Negative AV Hysteresis/ Search

The device decreases the AV delay by a programmed parameter when an intrinsic R wave is detected to encourage ventricular pacing. This remains in effect for 31 cycles after R-wave detection. If another R wave is not detected in that time, the permanently programmed AV delay is restored. If another R wave is detected during the 31-cycle period, the shortened AV delay remains in effect for 255 cycles.

65

Table 65.1 Manufacturer-Specific AV Hysteresis Programs (Continued)

BIOTRONIK

IOPT **AV Repetitive** **Hysteresis**	The AV delay is extended by a defined hysteresis value after sensing an intrinsic ventricular event for a programmed number of cycles. If an intrinsic rhythm occurs during one of the repetitive cycles, the long duration AV delay remains in effect. If an intrinsic rhythm does not occur during the repetitive cycles, the programmed AV delay resumes.
AV Scan Hysteresis	After 180 consecutive pacing cycles, the AV delay is extended for a programmed number of cycles. If an intrinsic rhythm is not detected within the number of scan cycles, the original AV delay value resumes.
Negative AV Delay **Hysteresis**	The AV delay is decreased by a defined value after a ventricular event is sensed, thereby promoting ventricular pacing. The normal AV delay resumes after the programmed number of consecutive ventricular paced events elapses.

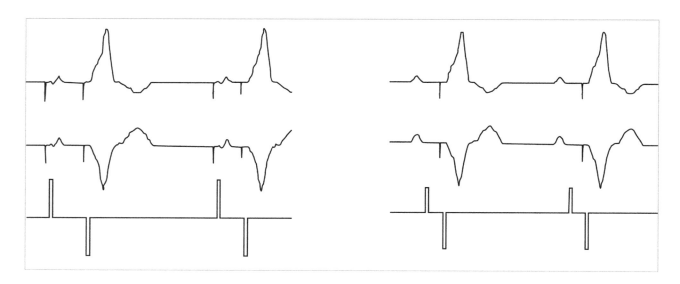

Figure 65.4 Atrial contraction.

A difference in the sensed and paced AV interval is routinely programmed to compensate for the latency between an atrial stimulus and actual atrial contraction (Figure 65.4). Right atrial leads are typically placed in the distal right atrial appendage (arrow, Figure 65.5). With atrial pacing, atrial electrical and mechanical activation occur at the time of pacing from the appendage, and the AP-VP interval is a true interval reflective of the timing between atrial and ventricular contraction. However, in sinus rhythm, the electrical wavefront starts in the region of the sinus atrial node, and by the time the wavefront reaches the atrial lead in the right atrial appendage, mechanical contraction of the atrium has already begun. Thus, the AS-VP interval is a pseudointerval and always shorter than the true AV contraction interval. To compensate for this difference, an offset is programmed—the differential AV interval.

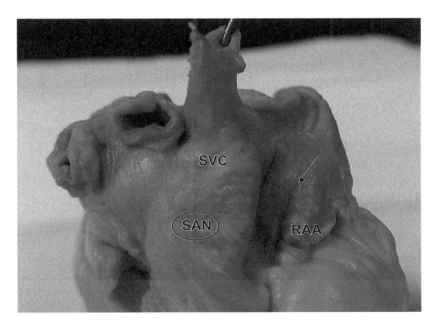

Figure 65.5 Location of atrial leads in the right atrial appendage (RAA). SVC = superior vena cava; SAN = sinus atrial node.

65

In the tracing in Figure 65.6, varying (progressively shortened) AV intervals are noted.

Rate-adaptive or dynamic AV interval shortens the sensed AV/positive AV at higher atrial rates (sinus tachycardia, sensor-driven atrial pacing) to mimic the physiological shortening of the PR interval at higher heart rates. The shortening of the AV interval also allows for a shorter TARP (Figure 65.7) at higher rates and decreases the likelihood of upper rate behavior.

Automatic PVARP (Medtronic) shortens the PVARP at higher pacing rates to prevent upper rate behavior (2:1 block). If the minimum programmed PVARP is reached and the heart rate is still higher, then the sensed AV is shortened to further decrease the TARP. Rate-adaptive AV interval and/or automatic PVARP would not explain the *longer* than expected AV delay noted in Figures 65.1 and 65.2.

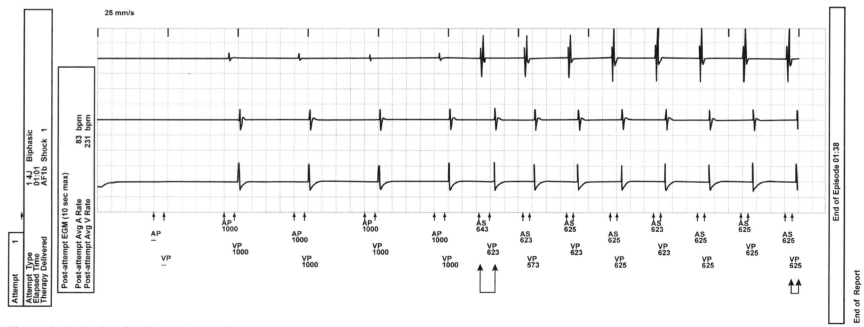

Figure 65.6 Tracing showing varying AV intervals.

65

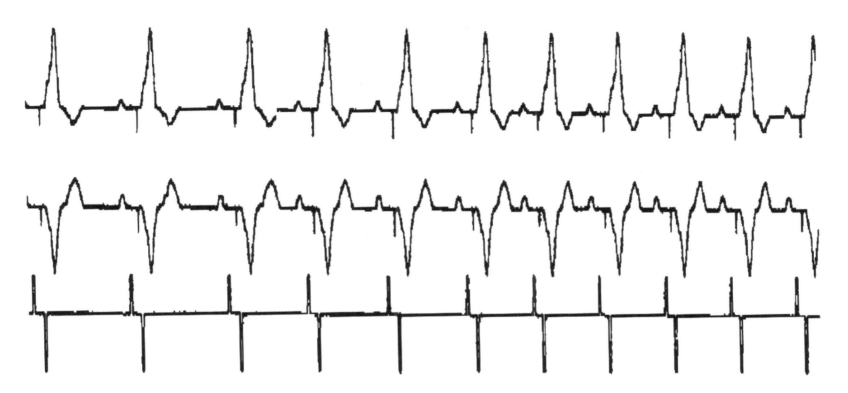

Figure 65.7 Shortening of the AV interval during pacing.

65

Figure 65.8 is obtained from a patient with a dual-chamber Medtronic pacemaker.

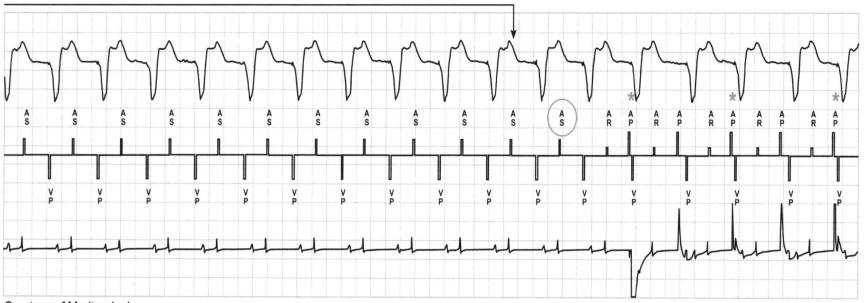

Courtesy of Medtronic, Inc.

Figure 65.8 Patient's tracing. Courtesy of Medtronic.

Q: *What is the likely cause of the very short AV intervals noted in Figure 65.8?*

1. Negative AV search hysteresis

2. Ventricular safety pacing

3. Noncompetitive atrial pacing

4. Managed ventricular pacing

65

3. Noncompetitive atrial pacing

Noncompetitive atrial pacing (NCAP, Medtronic) is intended to prevent induction of atrial fibrillation from atrial pacing occurring during the relative refractory period of the atrium. At the beginning of the tracing (Figure 65.8), we note pacemaker-mediated tachycardia (bracket) that terminates with extension of the PVARP leading to a retrograde atrial activation falling in the refractory period. If an atrial pacing stimulus is delivered too soon after the atrial refractory event, atrial tachycardia/fibrillation may be triggered. The atrial paced event if falling in the atrial absolute refractory period will not capture, and AV dyssynchrony may result. Several features are available in present devices to minimize these phenomena (A pace on PVC option, St. Jude Medical). With the NCAP feature, an atrial refractory event in the PVARP triggers a 300-ms interval (NCAP interval) during which no atrial pacing can occur, and the VA *interval is extended*. The pacemaker then attempts to maintain the lower rate by *shortening* the paced AV. Thus, a very short AV interval may be observed, as noted in Figure 65.8, leading to AV dyssynchrony for that cycle. In this case, the AP fails to capture, leading to repeat retrograde conduction and recurrent triggering of NCAP.

In addition to manifesting as unexpectedly short AV intervals, NCAP may also affect atrial and ventricular timing to produce a change in the paced rate compared to programmed parameters. If an atrial pacing stimulus is scheduled to occur during the NCAP period, the VA interval is necessarily extended until this period expires. The pacemak-

er will attempt to maintain a stable ventricular rate by shortening the paced AV, as noted; however, it will not shorten the paced AV to less than 30 ms. However, when higher lower rates and longer PVARPs are programmed, NCAP operation may result in ventricular pacing slightly below the lower rate.

Another situation where differences in AV intervals may be transiently observed occurs in conjunction with one of the available algorithms to assess adequacy of ventricular capture (capture management, etc.).

In Figure 65.9, a fusion avoidance algorithm associated with auto capture (St. Jude Medical) is diagrammed. Capture is assessed based on whether an evoked response (local EGM) can be sensed after the paced stimulus. At times, fusion from intrinsic conduction may mistakenly create the impression of failure to capture. To allow for this, the AV interval (in the Figure, a bracket) is extended by 100 ms to see if intrinsic conduction (fusion) is occurring and thus varying AV intervals may be noted on telemetry or a Holter monitor.

Managed Ventricular Pacing (MVP, Medtronic) (answer 4) is another algorithm intended to maximize intrinsic conduction.

In a transtelephonic transmission (Figure 65.10), the patient is initially paced AAI with intrinsic AV conduction occurring with a long AV interval (beats 1, 2). There is loss of AV conduction over the third atrial paced beat. Following this transient loss of AV conduction, the device

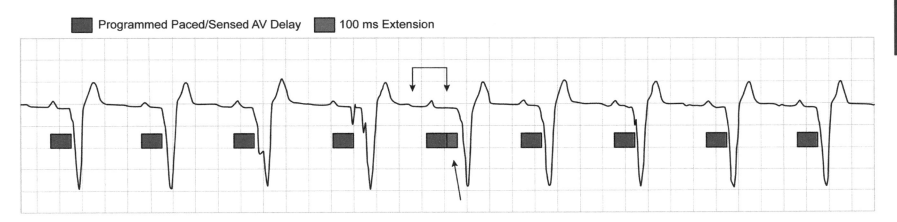

Figure 65.9 Fusion avoidance algorithm.

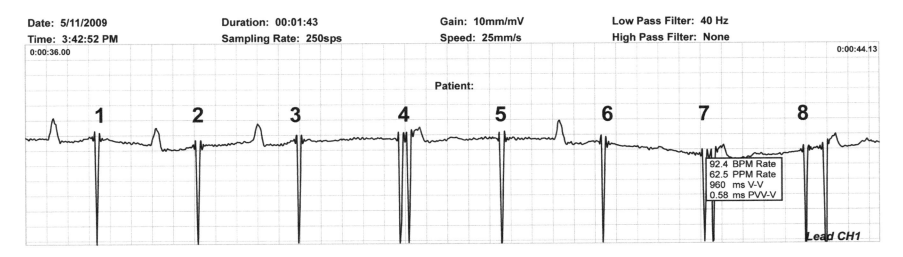

Figure 65.10 Patient's transtelephonic transmission.

65

delivers a backup ventricular pacing output with a *short* paced AV of 80 ms (beat 4). AAI pacing continues, and when beat 6 fails to conduct, the device delivers another backup ventricular pace (7). Persistent loss of AV conduction defined as the 2 most recent intervals missing a ventricular event is confirmed, and the device switches to DDD mode. The MVP algorithm may thus be associated with detected AV intervals different from the programmed parameters. Other features that may be noted on extended monitoring include:

- Periodic (1 min up to 16 h) single-cycle assessments of AV conduction, and resumption of AAI pacing
- Rarely in patients with 4:3 Wenckebach AV block, since every fourth beat is dropped and 2/4 are required for

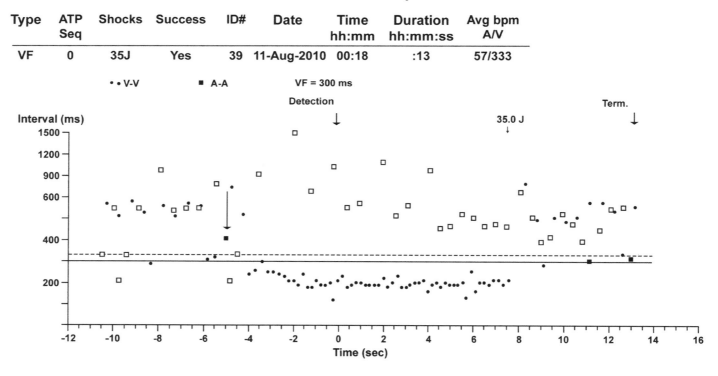

Figure 65.11 Treated VT/VF episode.

reversion to DDD pacing; continued AAI pacing with 4:3 block may continue

- Rarely, the variation in AV conduction and thus ventricular timing may be proarrhythmic (AVNRT induction from prolongation of atrial paced, ventricular sensed intervals) or in conjunction with frequent PVCs occasionally promoting ventricular arrhythmia (short-long-short sequences)

Figures 65.11 and 65.12 are obtained from a patient with abnormal repolarization (long QT syndrome). When switching from AAI to DDD pacing modes, variation in AV timing increased ectopy with further irregularity in ventricular activation promoting recurrent ventricular arrhythmia.

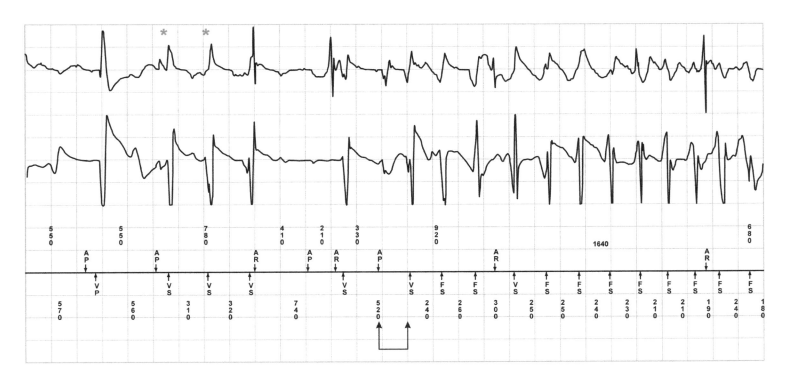

Figure 65.12 Increased ventricular ectopy.

65

When the patient was switched to AAIR pacing only (MVP off), the rhythm was stable with less PVCs and no ventricular arrhythmia (Figure 65.13). If AV conduction had been very poor, an alternate method could have been DDD pacing with a stable AV interval. This case, however, is an exception, and in most instances, algorithms such as AV search hysteresis or MVP allow assurance of ventricular activation when needed without unnecessary ventricular pacing.

Another cause of AV interval variability and discordant with programmed parameters is *negative* AV search hysteresis.

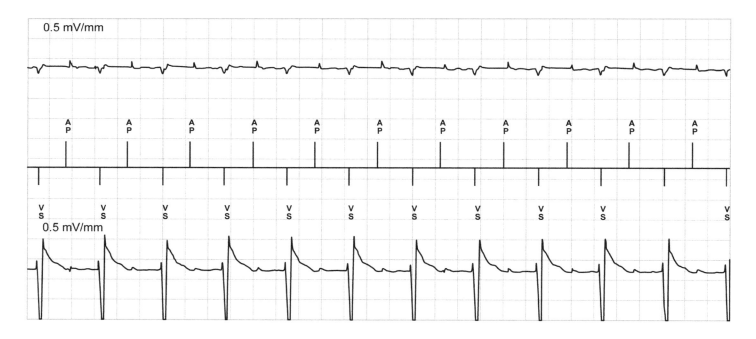

Figure 65.13 Reduced ectopy in AAI mode.

This algorithm is designed to promote ventricular pacing and prevent intrinsic conduct beats. In Figure 65.14, the programmed PVI and AVI are 150 ms and 175 ms, respectively. When intrinsic conduction occurs (AR), the AV interval is shortened with periodic lengthening of the AV interval (first arrow) to see if intrinsic conduction is no longer occurring and a relatively more physiological interval can continue. Negative AV search hysteresis may be useful with CRT devices and in patients with hypertrophic cardiomyopathy where the "pacing" is considered therapeutic and preferred to intrinsic conduction.

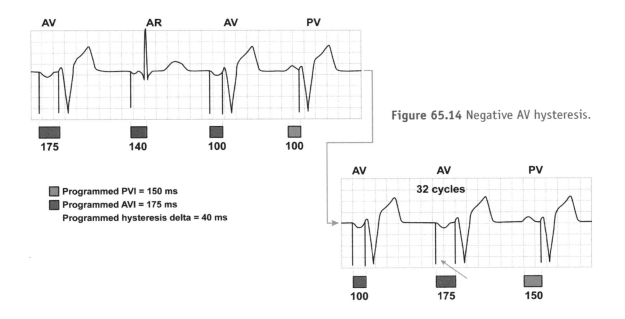

Figure 65.14 Negative AV hysteresis.

65

In Figure 65.15, initiation and termination of pacemaker-mediated tachycardia (PMT) is shown on a telemetry strip obtained from a patient with a dual-chamber pacemaker implanted 3 months ago for high-grade AV block. The patient presented with palpitation and was confirmed to have PMT.

Device settings:
- Mode: DDDR
- Pacing rate: 60 to 150 bpm
- AV delay: 100 ms; sensed AV delay: 100 ms
- PVARP: 250 ms
- Dynamic AV delay and AV search hysteresis: on

The device was reprogrammed to PVARP of 350 ms, and the upper tracking rate correspondingly decreased. However, as noted in this tracing, the patient continues to experience episodes of PMT.

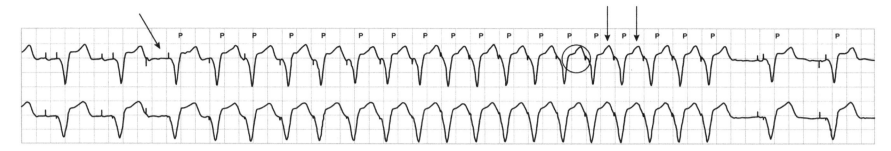

Figure 65.15 Patient's tracing.

Based on the observation in Figure 65.15, which of the following is the next best step in preventing future PMT episodes?

Q:

1. Increase PVARP further
2. Program off AV search hysteresis
3. Extend the PVAB
4. Program off dynamic AV delay

65

2. Program off AV search hysteresis

How does the episode of PMT start (arrow)? Note that there is an abrupt increase in the paced AV interval (AV search hysteresis). As a result, when ventricular pacing occurs, the AV node and atrium have recovered from refractoriness, and retrograde VA conduction may occur. This initiates PMT. Thus, limiting AV intervals, including by programming AV search hysteresis, will likely prevent such initiations.

Why does the PMT episode stop? There was likely automatic prolongation of the PVARP (PMT therapy) that terminated the episode. Also possible is retrograde VA block (see red arrows, likely retrograde P waves).

When frequent episodes of PMT are noted, a specific search for a proximate cause that allows VA conduction to occur should be made.

These triggers or associated features with frequent PMT include both patient-related and device-related causes. Patient-related causes include PVCs, PACs, the accessory pathway, and an interatrial conduction delay. Device-related causes include unusually short programmed PVARP, long programmed AV interval, atrial undersensing, and atrial failure to capture.

Pacemaker troubleshooting often involves close analysis of why AV intervals may be observed differently from programmed parameters. The rationale, mechanics, and, in some instances, pitfalls associated with algorithms that promote physiological AV synchrony should be understood, as illustrated by these cases.

65

Appendix

Spoiler alert! This appendix identifies the cases in this book by diagnosis, which may suggest or reveal the answers to questions in the cases. Because we want to encourage readers to approach the cases as unknowns, we are presenting this list as an appendix rather than as a table of contents and we recommend that you use the appendix only after working through the cases.

Index